Social-Emotional Learning
Starts with Us
Empowering Teachers to Support Students

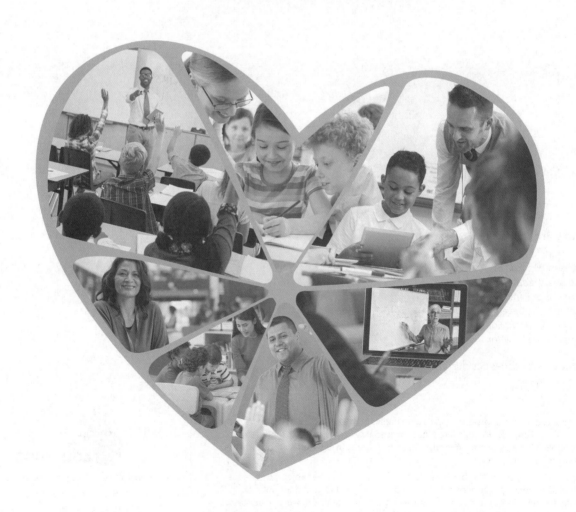

TRISHA DIFAZIO, M.A.T.
ALLISON ROESER, M.H.S.

Publishing Credits

Corinne Burton, M.A.Ed., *Publisher*
Aubrie Nielsen, M.S.Ed., *EVP of Content Development*
Véronique Bos, *Creative Director*
Cathy Hernandez, *Senior Content Manager*
Hillary Wolfe, M.A., *Developmental Editor*
David Slayton, *Assistant Editor*
Robin Erickson, *Art Director*

Image Credits: All images iStock and/or Shutterstock.

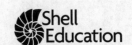

A division of Teacher Created Materials

5482 Argosy Avenue
Huntington Beach, CA 92649

www.tcmpub.com/shell-education

ISBN 978-1-0876-4918-4

© 2022 Shell Educational Publishing, Inc.
Printed in China 51497

Table of Contents

Table of Contents (cont.)

126898—Social-Emotional Learning Starts with Us

Foreword

It seems the term social-emotional learning (SEL) is everywhere these days—funny how a global pandemic, school closures, and social unrest can shift our priorities so dramatically. It's stunning to see how our perspectives on education have evolved more in one year—the first year of the pandemic—than in the previous 40 years. More than ever, we now realize that one of the most important components of education is to cultivate the social and emotional skills young people will come to rely on when faced with similar challenging events in their adult lives. All this to say: finally—we have arrived!

We are now at a place where we can move forward knowing that, from this point on, we *must* place as much value on SEL as on any other academic content area. In fact, academic learning cannot happen without social-emotional learning—they are not two separate things; they go hand in hand. Given the decades-long (that's right, SEL is not new!) body of research in support of SEL, we now know that the act of *learning*, in and of itself, is a social and emotional experience. Therefore, *all* learning is social and emotional in nature. This, coupled with the abundant science on how the brain functions in relation to how we learn, should have been a no-brainer (pun intended) all along. Nevertheless, we're here now.

The SEL world itself has evolved tremendously in recent years—like all good educators, we never stop learning! Still, even the SEL believers among us often struggle with what it is and how to teach it… which is why you're reading this book! The authors of *Social-Emotional Learning Starts with Us* are educators just like you, bringing you practical, real-world experiences and strategies you can apply in your own classrooms.

As educators, we are often reminded to remember our "why?" This means that when the stress of teaching (let's face it, teaching *is* stressful) gets to us, we stop, take a deep breath, and remind ourselves of *why* we went into teaching in the first place. What I've discovered in my 20-plus years in education is that teachers typically fall into one of two categories. Either they loved school as students themselves and have fond memories of their successful school experiences and want to *pay it forward*, or they're like me and, due to challenging life circumstances, found school to be irrelevant in preparing for the real world as an adult. Some kids from difficult backgrounds seek solace at school and thrive academically. Others are like me. They disengage and, in some cases, drop out altogether. The *why* for educators like me is the opportunity to change the life trajectory of students just like us.

Regardless of which category you fall into, or even if you don't relate to either one, we all need to remind ourselves from time to time of our *why*—which the authors invite you to reflect on in this book. Most of us in education are familiar with the research findings indicating how "one caring adult" in a child's life can have a dramatic and lifelong impact on a young person. That's why my motto is "Be the person you needed when you were young." Don't be afraid to be vulnerable with your students. Share with them the struggles and challenges you faced as a young person. This is how we connect with people of any age, on an emotional and personal level.

Just like us, kids must feel an emotional connection to their teacher to care about the content. It's as simple as that. The old adage still holds true—*They won't care how much you know until they know how much you care.*

Trisha DiFazio and Allison Roeser have a true passion for supporting educators and students. Simply put, they care. The fact that you're investing your time and energy in reading this book and in understanding why SEL must be a top priority says it all. You care too.

—Amy Cranston, Ed.D.
Executive Director, Social Emotional Learning
Alliance for California (SEL4CA) and author of
Creating Social and Emotional Learning Environments

Preface

Hi! We (Trisha and Allison) are so happy you are here! The purpose of this book is a simple one: to create connections. We're talking about connections in your brain, connections with others and most importantly—connecting with yourself. If you work in education, chances are you feel overwhelmed. We get it. We wrote this book for you. We want you to feel the same way your students do when they leave your class: supported, empowered, and inspired.

This book supports educators by providing a context for SEL in a way that actively involves all students and adults in developing their social and emotional skills. It also provides educators with a wide variety of SEL strategies and activities that can be easily integrated throughout the day or taught as stand-alone activities.

Inside, you will find personal inventories, reflection questions, captivating stories, educator and student spotlights, and differentiated grade-level appropriate SEL strategies and activities. Each activity, strategy, and tip in this book applies not only to your students, but to adults as well. This resource was designed to be flexible, so whether you'd like to learn solo or do a book study, this book has something for everyone.

In the **Introduction**, we define SEL, outline its long- and short-term benefits, and provide context for when and where it can be practiced. We examine the importance of adults developing their own social-emotional capacities before being able to effectively address those of students. We also explore the concept of *equity* and its relationship to SEL and consider the importance of leveraging SEL skills to provide equitable access to educational resources across race, gender, ethnicity, language, ability, sexual orientation, family background, and family income.

In the first five chapters, we look at the five core competencies of social-emotional learning. In **Chapter 1**, we identify and explore various facets of self-awareness, including understanding and labeling emotions, understanding identity, identifying cultural assets, having a growth mindset, recognizing strengths, and developing a sense of purpose. We start with the adult and then explore how those SEL skills can be applied in schools and classrooms. **Chapter 2** explores the concept of *self-management* and why it's important. We then focus on managing emotions, identifying stress, and setting goals while demonstrating personal and collective agency. We also offer several strategies to increase motivation in adults and students.

Social awareness is addressed in **Chapter 3**. We discuss the importance of understanding perspectives, seeking out resources, calling in support, practicing gratitude, and recognizing situational demands. We also include various suggestions for teaching, modeling, and building empathy. **Chapter 4** takes a deep dive into relationship skills and why they are essential. We provide strategies for how to develop positive relationships, connect across cultures, and create home-school connections. We offer simple and effective ways to connect and build trust with students and their families. In **Chapter 5**, we discuss why responsible decision-making is such an important skill to develop, not just for day-to-day but also for connecting to future goals. We explore the various contexts for responsible decision-making and provide multiple strategies with scaffolded support to aid students in this process. We also examine how reflection, ethics, and morals are incorporated into decision-making.

We have seen firsthand the power of mindfulness in supporting social-emotional learning, so **Chapter 6** focuses on this important concept. We discuss what mindfulness is and also what it is not. We also explore its many benefits for adults and children both in and outside the classroom. We provide helpful suggestions of how to integrate mindfulness practices, particularly breathing exercises, into instruction. We close the book with **Chapter 7**, where we have provided a collection of engaging SEL activities for grades K–12. This chapter starts with a chart showing which competencies are addressed in each activity. Each of the activities includes grade-level ideas, sentence frames, and multiple suggestions for differentiation.

About Us

We have been friends since high school and have both always been passionate about helping others. This passion is what led us both into education. Allison went into research, and Trisha went into the classroom. And while our lives have taken us to different cities over the years (Madrid; Washington, DC; Los Angeles; Chicago; San Francisco; and Baltimore), we'd spend hours catching up on the phone about all the things we were learning in our respective careers. We didn't realize this at the time, but a lot of what we were talking about was social-emotional learning. Combined, we have decades of experience in education, public health, mindfulness, professional coaching, and advocacy that we've drawn on to create this resource for you.

Allison

My parents like to tell a story about me in preschool: They say that at the end of the day, I would go up to each student in line and, one by one, help them zip up their jackets. Sometimes, I just did it myself. This is me in a nutshell. This passion for helping others is what fuels my work as a professional leadership coach, education consultant, and foster-youth advocate. I love all things that help people grow and develop.

My first job was designing leadership and life-skill curriculum for Chicago Public Schools. I would travel all over the city in my Honda Accord filled to the brim with athletic gear, crayons, snacks, and whatever else I was able to fundraise. It was a year of incredible growth and learning. This experience inspired me to get my master's degree in public health in hopes of impacting education on a large scale. What I realized later was that real change starts with the individual. For me, SEL offers skills and practical ways to create more ease in our lives. It's about understanding ourselves and each other. From my perspective, there is nothing better than supporting students and adults to live a life they are proud of.

Trisha

I love teaching. I started teaching because I wanted to be the teacher that I needed when I was young. In class, I was often bored or frustrated, preferring to chat or doodle instead of doing some worksheet. It wasn't until eighth grade that I met a teacher who finally understood how to engage me in learning. It was like I was being seen for the first time. As an adult, I wanted to pay that forward to kids. So, I became an ESL/Bilingual teacher (as it was called then). I was 22 years old and had no idea what I was doing. I made a ton of mistakes. Little did I know then that those mistakes would be some of the most profound learning experiences of my life. As we say in this book, mistakes grow our brain. It was during this time that I had a light bulb moment: How we feel impacts how we learn. I wanted to share this insight with as many educators as possible.

As a result, I became an adjunct professor of education at the University of Southern California, where I could focus on supporting and empowering educators. Additionally, I have spent the last ten years traveling around the country as an education consultant working directly with students, educators, and administrators. In that time, I've picked up many creative and engaging strategies from fellow educators, and I am happy to share them with you now.

As you can see, different paths have led each of us to this work. When we reflect on our own individual education experiences, we realize that it wasn't a worksheet or a PowerPoint that made a difference in our lives; it was a person. We designed this book for you to have a reflective, and maybe even transformative, experience. SEL starts with adults. SEL starts with us.

How to Use This Book

A few features have been called out to guide you in the learning process. Look for these sections as you read, and consider what they represent.

Quotation

Social-emotional learning impacts so many aspects of our lives. It is helpful to see how others have distilled these ideas into succinct nuggets of knowledge.

Personal Reflection

These questions help you think about your relationship to the content and its application to your own life.

Personal Inventory

These self-assessments support you in determining your strengths and areas for growth within each SEL competency.

Spotlight

Enjoy real-life stories and experiences from educators, experts, and students.

SEL in Action

Create opportunities throughout your day to integrate skill building and demonstrate SEL. These interactions offer ways to translate understanding into action for lasting impact on the culture of your classroom.

Storytime

Connect with us as we share our own real-life experiences.

Chapter Summary and Discussion Questions

Recall the major points of each chapter, and use these questions for personal reflection or as group discussion prompts.

Acknowledgments

First off, this book only exists because of the vision, support, and hard work of my dear friend and co-author, Allison Roeser. A huge thanks to my favorite teacher of all time, my wife Karen. I am so inspired by the work you do each and every day. I would also like to thank my parents for the emphasis they placed on education and the sacrifices they made to ensure that I received a quality one. Thank you, Dr. Eugenia Mora-Flores, for being the best possible mentor and friend. We are so grateful to Dr. Amy Cranston for her contribution to this book as well as her commitment to SEL. To all the teachers I have had the honor of working with over the years from District 89 Melrose Park-Maywood-Broadview, especially Mrs. Barb Dahly, thank you. Special thanks go out to Michelle DeLaRosa for her creativity and expertise. Last but not least, to all of my students over the years, you have been my greatest teachers. I am endlessly grateful. Thank you.

—Trisha

A special thanks to Trisha for including me in this work and bringing me "into the fold" to create this resource for educators. My heartfelt appreciation goes out to Sean, Nathan, and Luca for their constant support and always asking about the book at the dinner table. To my parents and siblings, your support over the years and your demonstration of SEL were the best lessons I ever could have asked for. To the Academy for Coaching Excellence for the training, wisdom, and tools to empower others. And always, to the students, educators, and fellow coaching colleagues—you challenge, support, and inspire me.

—Allison

Introduction

What Is Social and Emotional Learning?

We demonstrate social and emotional learning (SEL) skills without even knowing it, whether we are developing positive relationships or making a responsible decision. The point is, we all have some level of SEL skills already. We are here to help turn up the dial on what you already know—to support you in developing and practicing these skills for yourselves so that you can do the same for your students. The term *social and emotional learning* was coined by a group of researchers and educators in 1994. Their mission was to establish SEL as an essential part of K–12 education. Since then, the topic of SEL has become extremely popular—and for good reason.

The Collaborative for Academic, Social, and Emotional Learning (CASEL—pronounced *castle*) is an organization that supports educators and policy leaders to enhance experiences and outcomes for all students in grades pre-K–12. CASEL defines *SEL* as "an integral part of education and human development. SEL is the process through which all young people and adults acquire and apply the knowledge, skills, and attitudes to develop healthy identities, manage emotions and achieve personal and collective goals, feel and show empathy for others, establish and maintain supportive relationships, and make responsible and caring decisions" (CASEL, n.d.). SEL is not a content area, program, or product—it is a process. Its implementation both contributes to and depends upon an equitable learning environment where all students and adults feel respected, supported, and engaged.

CASEL 5

CASEL has identified five broad and interrelated competencies that include self-awareness, self-management, social awareness, relationship skills, and responsible decision-making. These are known as the *CASEL 5*. These competencies can be developed from childhood to adulthood and across various cultural contexts. As you can see from the CASEL Wheel (Figure 1.1), the competencies are interrelated, not hierarchical. There is also no endpoint. Just as a circle has no end, SEL is an ongoing process.

Figure 1.1: The CASEL Wheel

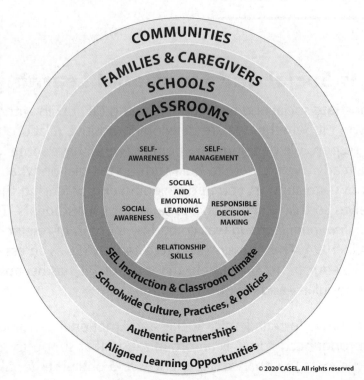

The CASEL Wheel represents a systemic approach. The rings around the CASEL 5 refer to the Key Settings, or the context in which these skills can be developed. The rings are included to emphasize the importance of establishing equitable learning environments. SEL is most beneficial when it is successfully integrated throughout the school's academic curricula and culture, across the broader contexts of schoolwide practices and policies, and through ongoing collaboration with families and community organizations.

In classrooms both virtual and in person, coordinated SEL efforts can foster youth voice, agency, and engagement. Enhanced adult SEL competence helps schools establish supportive classroom and school climates as well as supportive approaches to discipline. For families and caregivers, SEL is focused on establishing authentic family and community partnerships. In communities, organizations (e.g., before- and after-school programs, community-based organizations, health care providers, local businesses) that partner with schools can help foster alignment to the skills students are learning during the day and offer wraparound support. The frequency of SEL practices contributes to the culture of safety, inclusion, and belonging.

When and Where?

When and where can we practice SEL skills? The simple answer is *everywhere* and *all the time*. SEL skills can be developed as stand-alone lessons or activities like the ones we provide for each competency (see pages 109–161) and also what we call *SEL in Action*, meaning those instances in which SEL can be integrated and infused into your teaching practice. Sometimes, these are teachable SEL moments that deal with naming our emotions or resolving conflict, and other times, these might refer to practicing a self-management activity in times of stress. There are many opportunities to practice SEL skills on any given day.

SEL and State Standards

Standards are important because they give us a common language around SEL. They also demonstrate SEL as a priority worthy of our time, attention, and professional development. More and more states adopt SEL standards every year thanks in no small part to the 2015 Every Student Succeeds Act (ESSA) for highlighting the fact that "non-academic" indicators can also be used to measure student success. To learn more about your state's SEL standards, use the tool on the CASEL website (**casel.org/systemic-implementation/sel-policy-at-the-state-level/#know**).

Why SEL?

"Either we spend time meeting children's emotional needs by filling their love cup or we will spend time dealing with behaviors caused by their unmet needs. Either way we spend the time."

—Pam Leo (2007, 87)

In the past, the fields of child psychology and child development warned that too much love was dangerous for a child and would result in them being spoiled. However, current scientific research has taught us that children do best with demonstrative love and caring (Brackett 2019). Yep, the Beatles had it right: (Sing it with us!) *"All you need is (demonstrable) love (and caring)."* As a result, there is a great awakening taking place in education around SEL and it is this: a student's social and emotional well-being is essential to their learning. In an age of increased remote learning, we are witnessing districts, schools, and classrooms realizing the benefits of prioritizing the social and emotional well-being of their students—and staff! Turns out, it is all connected. We are all connected.

"You're not going to achieve the academic gains that you want to see without attending to the social and emotional development of young people."

—Karen VanAusdal, Senior Director of Practice for CASEL, (as cited in Barmore 2021, par. 36)

Another realization brought on by these challenging times is that it is more beneficial to be able to manage one's mind than to merely cram it with information. The days of rote memorization, drill-and-kill, or stand-and-deliver direct instruction are gone. "Sink-or-swim" approaches are not equitable, and they never have been. Why would we ever allow a child to sink?

As the world changes, our educational priorities shift and evolve. Recall, as a thinking skill, is no longer as important as it once was. After all, we have devices in our pockets that can recall every piece of information ever. As twenty-first century learners, our students need to be able to think creatively, work collaboratively, and to be innovative. These skills require taking risks, working well with others, and making mistakes. These skills require SEL.

Personal Reflection

What is your personal philosophy on making mistakes? How do you communicate that to your students?

You may wonder whether including SEL in the school day will take time away from the curriculum. Research shows the majority of academic learning does not happen until students feel safe and their social and emotional needs are met (Tennant et al. 2015; Kurtz et al. 2019).

 "The promotion of social, emotional, and academic learning is not a shifting educational fad; it is the substance of education itself. It is not a distraction from the 'real work' of math and English instruction; it is how instruction can succeed."

—Aspen Institute (2019, 6)

Recent advancements in neuroscience and education reveal just how strongly social and emotional skills influence all aspects of our lives. And if that is not compelling enough, a growing body of scientific evidence shows that social and emotional competencies in children and teens are *more* influential in determining major adult outcomes (such as health and financial success) than traditional metrics of academic success. SEL is not only effective at supporting development and improving outcomes in the moment, it can also act preventatively to minimize the likelihood of bullying, antisocial behavior, excessive risk-taking, anxiety, and depression (Center for Healthy Minds, n.d.).

Decades of research studies demonstrate the benefits of SEL, outlined in Figure 1.2.

Figure 1.2: Benefits of SEL

Short-Term	**Improved:** • attitudes about self, others, and tasks • perceptions of classroom and school climate
Intermediate	**Positive impacts on:** • social relationships and behaviors • academic success • classroom conduct • reduced emotional distress • reduced drug use
Long-Term	**Positive impacts on:** • high school graduation • college and career readiness • healthy relationships • mental health • reduced criminal behavior • civic engagement • safer sex decisions

Source: casel.org/wp-content/uploads/2020/08/CASEL-Equity-Insights-Report.pdf, p. 8

The Brain: Where It All Begins

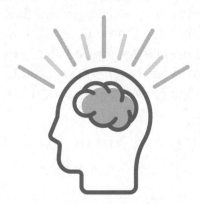

SEL is based on brain science that studies how human beings develop. What we know is that emotion and cognition are linked. Studies have shown that we think and learn best when we have supportive relationships, feel a sense of security and belonging, and have opportunities to process stress and emotions in healthy ways. Understanding the brain and how it works gives children and adults the opportunity to better understand their thoughts, emotions, and behaviors.

Advancing research sheds light on previously held ideas and beliefs about how our minds work. Recall the adage "You cannot teach an old dog new tricks." Well, it turns out that's not the case. Not only can you teach an old dog new tricks, but you can probably also teach it French. The human brain is a highly dynamic and constantly reorganizing system capable of being shaped and reshaped across an entire lifespan. Using what we know about the brain to our advantage, SEL can be a powerful process to support psychological development, academic growth, and overall well-being.

Thanks to one of the most exciting aspects of our brain—*neuroplasticity*—we can learn new things. *Neuroplasticity* refers to the brain's ability to adapt to changes in our environment by forming new neural connections over time. This means we have the potential to continue to learn new skills throughout our lives. When we learn something new, connections form between neurons and create new pathways in the brain. This is great news for all of us, so why not share this information with your students? Explain to them that the brain changes and grows as they learn and that they can get better at a skill by trying, practicing, and persevering.

"When our brains and bodies perceive threat, we protect and defend through our behaviors. When we are fear-filled, angry, anxious, or worried, our nervous systems are not available for learning, reasoning, logic or rewards, stickers, and consequences."

—Dr. Lori Desautels (2021)

Our "Why"

We wrote this book to empower educators and students.

Our "why" is that SEL speaks to the heart of what it is to be human. SEL reminds us that the abilities to resolve conflict, manage emotions, and effectively problem-solve are skills that can improve through practice. We truly believe that once you start to practice SEL skills consistently, you will experience more ease in your life, whether in remote learning or in a classroom—and yes, even in your personal relationships. It is the same for our students. SEL skill development is a lifelong journey. So, wherever you find yourself in your personal journey, we are happy to accompany you for this part.

Spotlight

For high school principals, the transition to distance learning meant tackling a lot of logistical issues. That is just one facet of the administrator's job; the other is the human element. In times of crisis, we need connection. It was imperative that my teachers felt supported, personally and professionally. Before we could attend to the SEL needs of our students, I knew I needed to attend to the SEL needs of my teachers. I brought in an SEL consultant and we dove into the learning as a team. As a participant, I noticed that the staff learned about and connected with each other. These SEL sessions really supported all of us in developing our personal SEL skills. The results were amazing. At the end of the day, the well-being of my team affects our students and is critical to our success as a school.

—Stacey Honda
Principal, Schurr High School
Montebello, California

Personal Reflection

What is your "why" when it comes to SEL? Why is it important to you?

SEL Starts with Adults

Teaching can be stressful. You know it. We know it. Science knows it. In fact, teaching has been recognized as one of the most stressful jobs in the United States (Herman, Hickmon-Rosa, and Reinke 2018; Lopez and Sidhu 2013). In one study, Herman found that more than 9 in 10 elementary school teachers feel high levels of stress (Herman, Hickmon-Rosa, and Reinke 2018, 96). What if we told you that your ability to take care of yourself is an invaluable part of your students' success? According to Herman, "we as a society need to consider methods that create nurturing school environments not just for students, but for the adults who work there" (News Bureau, University of Missouri 2018.)

We could not agree more. For students to succeed, we need to focus on the well-being of educators. There is a myth that SEL is for younger children and younger children only. This couldn't be further from the truth. SEL skills benefit everyone. Think about it: if SEL is designed to support students with their social and emotional health and improve well-being, wouldn't we want the same for ourselves?

As educators, we cannot teach what we do not know. To be the most effective teachers, administrators, and support staff, we must first understand and then develop our own social-emotional capacities before we can address those of our students. SEL starts with adults. That is why this book begins with *you*. Much of what we understand of the world comes from our mindset. Our brains filter information through a prism of our own experiences. Our mindset impacts our behavior and influences how we interact with others.

Quality SEL instruction occurs when educators are emotionally aware. Emotionally aware educators are more adaptive, resilient, and better able to connect to their students. As a result, you are an integral part of creating a classroom environment for students to thrive. Not only will this understanding of SEL increase the quality of relationships with your students and colleagues, but it will also contribute to *your* overall sense of well-being. This resource is going to guide you in successfully implementing SEL strategies while looking at how to foster your own emotional awareness with support and create community around SEL engagement.

Whether you are an SEL expert or a novice, we appreciate you. You do the hard work of shaping our youth as well as the "heart" work. If we were Oprah Winfrey, this is the part where we would give you a mid-sized sedan (You get a car!). While we cannot gift you a vehicle, we can offer you this book—a guide to support you in developing your SEL skills. Now, we know you do not need one more thing on your plate. As referenced in Amy Cranston's *Creating Social and Emotional Learning Environments* (2019), Gene Olsen states, "SEL is not one more thing on your plate; it is the plate" (68).

Personal SEL Inventory

Taking stock of where you are with each competency will serve as a springboard for what's next in your SEL learning. Now, let's take a little inventory of your own proficiency in the five SEL competencies. Read the descriptions in the first column, and put a check mark in the column that best describes you.

Self-Awareness

	I don't know what you're talking about.	I'm on my way, but could use a little help.	I'm pretty good at this.	I'm awesome at this.
I know my strengths and areas for growth.				
I know my various identities (e.g., racial, ethnic, gender).				
I actively engage in examining my bias.				
I believe intelligence can be improved through dedication and hard work.				
I am aware of my emotions.				

Self-Management

	I don't know what you're talking about.	I'm on my way, but could use a little help.	I'm pretty good at this.	I'm awesome at this.
I know how to set meaningful goals in my life.				
I can identify personal sources of stress.				
I can effectively manage my emotions.				
I know what I can do to help myself when I'm stressed/I practice self-care.				
I practice mindfulness/ know how to use breathing strategies to reduce stress.				

Social Awareness

	I don't know what you're talking about.	I'm on my way, but could use a little help.	I'm pretty good at this.	I'm awesome at this.
I understand and model empathy.				
I consider other people's perspectives during an interaction.				
I practice gratitude daily.				
I validate students' home language.				
I validate cultures that are different from my own.				

Relationship Skills

	I don't know what you're talking about.	I'm on my way, but could use a little help.	I'm pretty good at this.	I'm awesome at this.
I communicate effectively with others.				
I offer support to others easily.				
I seek support from others easily.				
I stand up for the rights of others.				
I prioritize building positive relationships with all of my students.				

Responsible Decision-Making

	I don't know what you're talking about.	I'm on my way, but could use a little help.	I'm pretty good at this.	I'm awesome at this.
I evaluate options before making a decision.				
I demonstrate curiosity and open-mindedness when making a decision.				
I support students in evaluating the consequences of their decisions.				
I consider how institutions impact individuals and communities.				
I consider how the decisions I make will impact others.				

Personal Reflection

Take a look at where most of your check marks fall. Do you notice any patterns? What did you learn about yourself from the inventory? What surprised you?

The Negativity Bias

Have you ever noticed how easy it is to focus on what is "wrong" with a situation or what *might* go wrong? For example, one of our SEL webinars was posted on YouTube®. While we were so excited when it reached 100 "likes," we were fixated on the one "dislike." We talked about it for weeks. Did fixating on the one dislike serve us in any way? No, of course not. We just kept running this script in our minds where we questioned ourselves, our teaching, and even our worthiness. Wow, that escalated quickly.

Is an experience like this familiar to you? If so, you are not alone! It is called the *negativity bias*. The *negativity bias* is a psychological term used to describe how negative things have a greater effect on us than neutral or positive things. It is an evolutionary phenomenon. Picture it now: you live in a cave. You are hungry. You venture out for food, and the moment the sunlight hits your toe, what is the first thing you look for? That's right, you look for danger. We are descendants of people who were very good at looking for danger and anticipating what could go wrong. It kept us alive! Believe it or not, our brains have not changed much since we were living in caves. Fast-forward to today: our brain does not make a distinction between the stress of running from a predator and the stress and excitement of a job interview. The triggers of stress have evolved but not the science of how our body responds.

Research has shown people tend to focus more on the negative. For example, we tend to:

- remember traumatic experiences better than positive ones
- recall insults better than praise
- react more strongly to negative stimuli
- think about negative things more frequently than positive ones
- respond more strongly to negative events than to equally positive ones (Cherry 2020)

Negativity Bias and Learning

Given that negativity bias is a natural human tendency, we can unintentionally operate from this bias when perceiving and interacting with others. Specifically, this bias can have a large impact on our relationships with students because our brains are primed to focus on negative behaviors.

As educators, if we have 10 interactions with a student and nine are positive, it is likely our brain will focus more on the one that was negative. How could focusing on a negative interaction affect your perception of that student? For adults, there is much to be gained by seeing how the negativity bias impacts interactions with students, staff, administrators, parents, and community members.

 # Personal Reflection

Where have you noticed the negativity bias in your experience as an educator?

Now, we've seen "behind the curtain" and understand the brain's natural tendency to slant toward the negative. From this moment forward, we have a choice. We can choose to focus on what's going right or wrong. One powerful way to do this is to shift our attention from focusing on deficits to focusing on assets. When we practice self-awareness and self-management skills, we can see situations more clearly. It is also important to note that the opposite of the negativity bias is *not* positive thinking. We must acknowledge when things are challenging, but we can choose to focus our attention on skillfully managing our responses. When we can do that, we are better able to have constructive conversations, provide constructive feedback, or even share negative emotions with more ease and productivity.

Equity

What Is Equity?

Educational equity occurs when "every student has access to the educational resources and rigor they need at the right moment in their education across race, gender, ethnicity, language, disability, sexual orientation, family background and or/family income." (Schlund, Jagers, and Schlinger 2020). While *equality* means treating every student the same, *equity* means making sure every student has the support they need to be successful. Basically, *equality* is making sure every kid gets a pair of shoes for the race, *equity* is making sure they have the right size. Ultimately, equity is about all students having access to what they need to be successful in school.

 "For all students to benefit, SEL must be grounded in a larger context of equity and justice efforts within public education. Doing so will help to identify and dismantle barriers that prevent many students from accessing and benefitting from SEL."

—Dena N. Simmons, Marc A. Brackett, and Nancy Adler (2018)

Spotlight

What do I wish my teacher knew? I wish my teacher knew that I have to catch the bus to get to school, and I don't always have the fare. When I walk, there are some neighborhoods I have to avoid for my safety. I wish my teacher knew that when I show up to class late, I need help, not punishment. I wish my teacher knew that if I fall asleep in class it's because it's loud where I live, and it makes it hard to sleep at night. I wish my teacher knew that I act tough in class so that my classmates don't mess with me. I wish my teacher knew that I'm not trying to disrespect them, I'm just trying to stay safe.

—Marie Greenwood
Former Student, Locke High School
Watts, California

Equity and SEL

We cannot talk about SEL without discussing its relationship to equity. However, this wasn't always the case. There was a time in SEL's development when it did not include terms like *cultural competence* and *equity*, which begged the question of whether the earlier version of SEL was truly beneficial for *all* students. The COVID-19 pandemic seems to have fast-tracked America's long overdue reckoning with inequities across multiple systems throughout our nation, especially education.

The pandemic, and the subsequent shift to remote learning for many schools, magnified many of the problems that existed during in-person school. If teaching practices didn't meet the needs of students in traditional in-person classes, how could they meet the needs of students remotely? Especially considering those students who rely on school for free and reduced lunch or access to the internet, among other things. SEL is at its strongest when it is leveraged as a strengths-based approach that affirms and promotes understanding of diverse identities, strengths, values, lived experiences, and cultures. A culturally responsive approach, one that situates and celebrates learning within the rich cultural contexts of students, may be the key to bridging this gap and ensuring that all students can reap the full benefits of SEL instruction (Irvine and Hawley 2011; Ladson-Billings 1994).

SEL alone cannot combat all the problems of society nor can it solve long-standing and deep-seated inequities. It can, however, be used as a lever for equity by helping schools "promote understanding, examine biases, reflect on and address the impact of racism, build cross-cultural relationships, and cultivate adult and student practices that close opportunity gaps and create a more inclusive school community. In doing so, schools can promote high-quality educational opportunities and outcomes for all students, irrespective of race, socioeconomic status, gender, sexual orientation, and other differences" (CASEL 2022).

We can support SEL as a level for equity when we:

- offer instruction that affirms the dignity and humanity of all people
- advocate for curriculum that is inclusive
- implement curriculum that not only includes but also champions the diverse experiences of people across cultures
- provide opportunities and routines that reinforce skills, habits, and mindsets
- incorporate culturally competent asset-based approaches
- include and examine issues and events from multiple perspectives
- provide identity-safe classrooms where everyone's story is not only recognized but honored

As stated earlier, SEL, as a field of study, is ever evolving. CASEL is currently refining a specific form of SEL implementation called *Transformative SEL* that intentionally and specifically concentrates SEL practice on transforming inequitable settings and systems and promoting justice-oriented civic engagement. CASEL defines *Transformative SEL* as "a process whereby young people and adults build strong, respectful, and lasting relationships that facilitate co-learning to critically examine root causes of inequity, and to develop collaborative solutions that lead to personal, community, and societal well-being." While Transformative SEL research is underway, equity is woven throughout the strategies and activities in this book.

Summary

SEL starts with adults. As educators, we want to be able to model the SEL skills that we are seeking to develop in our students. A deeper understanding of the brain and awareness of our mindset tells an optimistic story about the potential we all have as learners. Now that you have completed the inventory, you have a better idea of where you are and where you're headed in your SEL journey.

Like us, SEL wasn't born fully formed; it has grown and developed over time. The arc of SEL bends toward a more just, inclusive, equitable learning experience for all students and teachers. All students deserve equal access to SEL skills and equitable learning environments where they feel respected, supported, and engaged.

Discussion Questions

1. What are your biggest takeaways from this section?

2. How can you apply the knowledge you have gained from this section?

3. What aspects of SEL are you interested in learning more about?

Chapter 1: Self-Awareness

What Is Self-Awareness?

> "If only I had checked myself."
> —guy who wrecked himself

OK, it is not exactly Socrates, but you get the point. As we have said before, we cannot teach beyond where we have gone ourselves. For that reason, cultivating self-awareness is as beneficial for *you* as it is for your students. The more self-aware an educator is, the more capable they are of creating high-quality social and emotional learning environments.

CASEL defines *self-awareness* as "the ability to understand one's own emotions, thoughts, and values and how they influence behavior across contexts." This includes capacities to recognize one's strengths and limitations with a well-grounded sense of confidence and purpose. For example, one who is self-aware can:

- identify emotions
- integrate personal and social identities
- identify personal, cultural, and linguistic assets
- have a growth mindset
- recognize one's strengths and areas of growth
- develop interests and sense of purpose
- demonstrate honesty and integrity
- link feelings, values, and thoughts
- examine prejudices and biases

Why Is Self-Awareness Important?

Becoming more self-aware helps us to manage our thoughts, emotions, and behaviors rather than allowing them to manage us. The more self-aware we are, the better able we are to *feel* hurt without *spreading* hurt. Intentionally working to become more self-aware helps us to show up in the classroom (and the world) as the best versions of ourselves. Wouldn't a dose of self-awareness make a family holiday dinner better for most of us? So, why isn't everyone running out to become a self-awareness expert? Good question. Self-awareness is an "inside job," and it requires a fair amount of self-exploration, which can be uncomfortable at times. The beauty of self-awareness is that once you discover something about yourself, you cannot undiscover it. Until now, many of us simply have not had the support to develop and practice this skill. But do not despair—as previously mentioned, with neuroplasticity, it is never too late to learn.

Identifying One's Emotions

This one goes out to our English teachers—we know how much you love Greek and Latin roots! The word *emotion* comes from the Latin *e*, meaning "out," and *movere*, meaning "to move." Emotions are meant to move through us. Babies are a great example of how to exhibit emotional health—they let their emotions come and go; feelings pass through them like clouds moving through the sky.

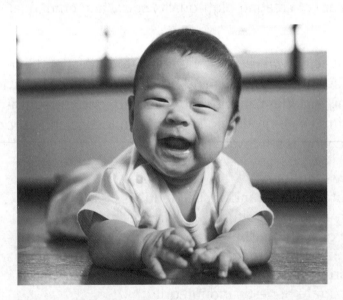

It is not until later in life that we learn to hold on to, hide, or suppress our emotions. The reality is that emotions are neither good nor bad. We learn about emotions from observations of those around us. In that regard, our culture has a big influence on how we learn to express, demonstrate, and regulate our emotions. Emotions are vital pieces of information. However, most of us were never taught how to recognize our emotions or to consider the important messages they carry. With time and practice, we can get better at knowing what we are feeling and why. Identifying and managing our emotions help us to evaluate our response so we can control our emotions rather than the emotions controlling us. We often see students getting swept away in a whirlwind of their emotions, especially during puberty. And if you find yourself getting frustrated with a student's behavior, we invite you to remind yourself of one of our favorite quotes: "Emotional regulation is not instinctive; it is learned" (Maynard and Weinstein 2019).

There are no "bad" kids, just young people expressing their wants and needs the only way they know how. Children who do not learn to regulate their emotions become adults who have difficulty regulating their emotions. Unfortunately, society has a lot less empathy for adults with poor emotional regulation. It is easy to blame parents for their children's behavior, but oftentimes these parents also never learned the necessary skills to teach and model for their children, thus creating a cycle.

 # Personal Reflection

What types of classroom management practices did you experience as a student? How were emotions handled in the classroom?

There are many current classroom management systems that disregard or disapprove of emotion, offering only punitive measures rather than the necessary guidance needed to resolve the situation. However, when a child is criticized for expressing his or her emotions (e.g., crying, yelling), it can lead to an even more intense demonstration of that emotion (Maynard and Weinstein 2019).

In SEL, we prioritize responding over reacting. A large part of SEL is being able to effectively name and manage emotions. These emotions originate in the brain. When we can label an emotion, we can create a distance between ourselves and our experience that allows us to choose how we respond rather than simply reacting to challenges. Based on research using magnetic resonance imaging, we now know that the simple act of labeling an emotion makes it less intense (Hammond 2015). This act of labeling an emotion is a form of regulation. We are most vulnerable to the impact of emotions that we fail to detect and understand. For this reason, having an emotional vocabulary is an excellent way to help us label and manage emotions.

Most of our greetings and check-ins with people are on autopilot: "How are you?" elicits an automatic "I'm fine" response (even when we aren't fine).

 ## SEL in Action

What's Your Battery Life?

This strategy is a great way to gauge overall energy levels of adults and students to better know how they are really doing. Simply ask what their current battery life is on a scale from 0 percent to 100 percent. Whether they report being at 5 percent or 99 percent, it gives us a helpful insight that will inform our interactions moving forward.

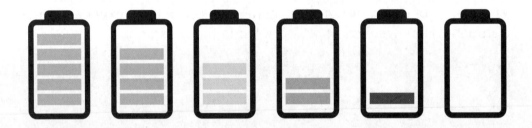

Put It on a Scale

This important self-assessment strategy helps adults and students evaluate the intensity of their feelings. In other words, it helps to determine how "big" emotions are. Understanding this nuance is empowering and will help us more clearly understand what we are experiencing. As a result, we can then articulate our needs more effectively to one another. Here are a few examples for students.

PreK–2nd grade students: You can ask, "Is this a small, medium, or large [*insert feeling*]?"

3rd–12th grade students: You can ask, "On a scale from 1 to 10, how [*insert feeling*] are you?"

You can also do "fist to five," where students use their fingers to indicate on a scale from 0 to 5 how well they understand a topic or how excited they are about something. Mix and match scales to do whatever fits your class best. The most important part is to give yourself and your students the opportunity to self-assess.

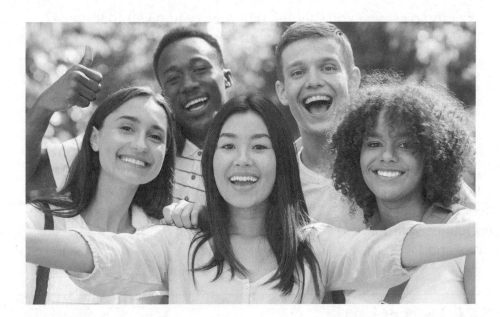

Identity

We all have multiple identities. The sense of self for young people is informed by these identities, including, for example, cultural values and orientations as well as collective identities such as ethnic-racial group, socioeconomic status, and gender (Jagers et al. 2018). Students feel safe, accepted, and valued when they can share their identities with their teachers and classmates. In that regard, self-awareness is foundational for equity. We want our students to know that they do not have to lose, deny, or leave any element of their identities or their culture at the door to achieve success.

We are better able to support students in understanding their personal and social identities when we understand our own. There are entire books and courses dedicated to this topic—and for good reason. The concept of identity is complex and highly nuanced. The bottom line is: our role is to support students to discover and tell us who they are—not to assign them identities.

We all want to cultivate a classroom climate that is equitable and fair to all students and their identities. Knowing our students' names and how to pronounce them correctly is one of the first steps in creating a positive classroom culture. This conveys these important messages: I care about you, I accept you, and you are important to me. Instead of calling students out individually, here are a few questions you can pose to all your students to get to know them:

- Who gave you your name? Why were you given that name?
- Do you know the origin of your name?
- Do you have any nicknames? If so, how did you get them?
- What is your preferred name?
- How do you pronounce your name?
- What pronouns do you use?

If you have difficulty learning or saying a student's name, do not be afraid to ask. It is always better to be curious than to assume. One option is having all your students teach you their names when you meet them. For example: "It is important to me that I learn and pronounce your names correctly. So, let me know how you say your name, and I'll do my best to say it correctly."

 # SEL in Action

Show your students that you take pronouncing their names seriously. Here are a few tips to help:

The first time you meet	• Repeat the name a few times. • Note how to phonetically pronounce the name.
The first few days of school	• Continue to ask as necessary. (Avoid asking publicly.) It is OK if you have to respectfully ask them a couple of times. • For example, say, "It is important to me that I say your name correctly. Can you please remind me how to pronounce your name again?" • Apologize if you get it wrong. For example, say, "I'm sorry I mispronounced that. Could you please repeat your name for me?"
Every day thereafter, and especially around others	• Be mindful not to emphasize your difficulty pronouncing the student's name. When this happens it becomes about the adult and their difficulty, which inadvertently makes it the student's problem.

Storytime

During one professional development session, we were discussing the importance of pronouncing a student's name correctly. A student's name, like their home language and home culture, is essential to his or her identity.

I posed the question, "What would keep us from saying our students' names correctly?"

One participant raised his hand and said, "It is hard because a lot of my students have 'made-up' names."

Think about that statement for a moment. What did he mean by "made-up names"? We proceeded to have an in-depth conversation. He realized that regardless of the name, all names are essentially "made up." His students' names were not too difficult for him to learn; they were merely culturally unfamiliar to him.

 # Personal Reflection

Have you ever had your name mispronounced? How did that make you feel? Have you ever been in a situation where you mispronounced a students' name? Moving forward, what could you do differently?

Identifying Cultural and Linguistic Assets

The lens through which we view our students impacts how we treat them. If we look through a deficit lens, we will perceive what they *do not* have rather than what they *do* have. We cannot build on deficits; we can only build on assets. It is the difference between building a house on a solid foundation versus quicksand. Each student brings with them a wealth of lived experiences that are deeply rooted in their language and culture. When we understand that these experiences are assets and not deficits, we become more culturally responsive. "Culturally and Linguistically Responsive Teaching and Learning (CLR) is the validation and affirmation of indigenous (home) culture and language with the purpose of building and bringing the students into success in the culture of academia and mainstream society." (Hollie 2018). When we validate and affirm students around essential aspects of their identities, like their languages and cultures, they feel seen, heard, and valued.

Language and culture are essential to our identities. Building meaningful relationships with all students means understanding who they are at their core. Stakeholders who are culturally responsive create more meaningful, sustaining connections with students. Culturally Responsive Practices (CRP) (Ladson-Billings 2014; Gay 2000) provide an important asset-based lens through which educators can implement SEL in effective, equitable ways. The most powerful educational experiences occur when students' identities, cultures, and experiences are elevated as assets. Why? It all comes back to the brain. "It is about engaging the brain's memory systems and information processing structures so we're creating lessons that lean into students' cultural traditions and values, allowing them to learn in ways that are uniquely suited to them" (Hammond 2015).

Any language you use to tell your mom, grandma, or brother that you love them is legitimate. Linguistically, students come to school with various levels of English and home-language proficiency. Regardless of those levels, all home languages are legitimate. We cannot meet the social and emotional needs of students if we are telling them that the way they speak at home is wrong, broken, or bad. Students learning English as a second language and students who speak English in a nonstandard way are often being viewed through a deficit lens. This results in teachers overcorrecting them rather than focusing on the linguistic capabilities they already have.

Bilingual and multilingual students should be walking around school with their heads held high because they can speak more than one language. When stakeholders lift up their bilingual students by praising and validating their abilities, they help counter this dangerous narrative that being bilingual is somehow shameful. When we show and tell our students that we are proud of them, it helps them to be proud of themselves. This sense of pride contributes to their personal agency.

You do not need to become an expert on all cultural groups and languages. However, it is important to understand your students' cultural and linguistic identities to create relevant learning opportunities and make instructional decisions that reflect the experiences and values of our students. In the words of Ted Lasso, "Be curious, not judgmental." When in doubt, you can simply ask students about themselves and their families.

Spotlight

The connection between language and social-emotional learning is strong! One cannot happen without the other. It is not about one coming before or after, but that language development practices and SEL work side by side simultaneously. For decades, the literature on second language acquisition shared the importance of students learning in environments that felt safe and supportive to take risks with language. If students do not feel engaged and ready to learn, it can limit their opportunities for learning. After over 20 years of working with teachers in language development for all learners K–12, across all curricular areas, I am often reminded of the need to share this synergistic relationship between language and SEL. When I walk into classrooms and see students nervous to speak or afraid to make mistakes, I remember how hard it was to learn language and content at the same time. Without the support from peers and teachers that believed in me, I would have never gained the confidence to take risks, and in turn, succeed academically.

—Dr. Eugenia Mora-Flores
Professor of Education
University of Southern California

Having a Growth Mindset

The concept of a *growth mindset* was developed by psychologist Carol Dweck and popularized in her book *Mindset: The New Psychology of Success*. Dweck focuses on the difference between *fixed* and *growth* mindsets. In a *fixed mindset*, people believe that their basic qualities, like their intelligence or talent, are simply traits that can't change. Whereas in a *growth mindset*, people believe that their most basic abilities can be developed through dedication and hard work. If you have a growth mindset, it "creates a love of learning and a resilience that is essential for great accomplishment" (Dweck 2006). Yes, please! I'll take one of those.

Mindset Inventory

Since SEL starts with us, let's check in on our mindsets. Do you currently have a growth or a fixed mindset? Let's find out! Put a check mark next to each question that you would answer with a yes. Which mindset most accurately describes you?

Fixed Mindset: Do you...	**Growth Mindset: Do you...**
☐ give up easily when things get hard?	☐ persevere despite challenges?
☐ fear making a mistake?	☐ see mistakes as a valuable way to learn?
☐ ignore feedback or take it personally?	☐ solicit and stay open to feedback?
☐ stick only to what you know?	☐ feel excited to learn new things?
☐ think skills are something you're born with? (You either "have it" or you don't.)	☐ think skills come with hard work and can always develop?
☐ get discouraged and blame others when experiencing a setback?	☐ view setbacks as opportunities to improve next time?

The difference between fixed and growth mindsets has far-reaching implications for educators and students. What makes the growth mindset so profound is that it creates a passion for learning rather than a hunger for approval. People with growth mindsets are not discouraged by failure. In fact, they do not even see themselves as failing in those situations—they see themselves as learning.

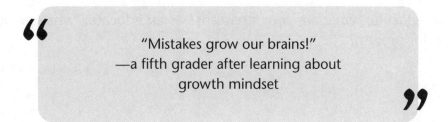

"Mistakes grow our brains!"
—a fifth grader after learning about
growth mindset

Recognizing One's Strengths and Areas for Growth

You might notice that we changed the word *limitations* in CASEL's definition to *areas for growth*. We did so because we believe the term *areas for growth* is best aligned with a growth mindset. There are several ways to think about one's strengths. Personally, reflecting on your strengths and areas for growth as an educator is a great start. However, it is not the whole kit and caboodle. We can only see so much when reflecting on our own. One of the fastest ways to discover and identify strengths and areas for growth is through feedback.

There is tremendous value in hearing from people you trust and who know you well; they often shine a light on a strength or skill you have taken for granted or simply do not see. As a result, this section addresses your personal reflections as well as feedback solicited from colleagues and students.

Opening up to others to ask these types of questions can make you feel vulnerable, but it is also a great opportunity to demonstrate a growth mindset. Here, we can practice what we preach! We all have areas for growth—it is a natural and normal part of human development. However, sometimes our thoughts can get in a mental tangle. Maybe we take something personally or take feedback out of context. Before we know it, we are so busy tending to our "upset" that we have completely lost the golden nugget of the feedback. If that sounds like a familiar experience, try using a growth mindset on for size and see if the process becomes slightly more enjoyable. We invite you to participate in this three-part process to get a more comprehensive understanding of your strengths and areas for growth as an educator. Warning: You might be pleasantly surprised to see what your students and colleagues appreciate about you.

Personal Reflection

As an educator, what are your strengths? As an educator, what are your areas for growth?

Colleague Feedback

Choose a trusted colleague, and ask them the following questions:

1. As an educator, what do you see as my strengths?

2. As an educator, what do you see as my areas for growth?

Student Feedback

Have students answer these questions:

1. In the classroom, what helps you learn?

2. In the classroom, what makes it hard for you to learn?

3. What do you want to do more of in class?

4. What do you want to do less of in class?

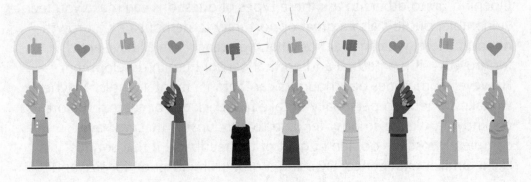

"If we are not asking them what they need, we are not giving them what they need."

—Dena Simmons (2019)

In terms of our teaching, our students are extremely valuable assets in helping us cultivate more self-awareness. When we asked students the above questions, these were some of the responses. (Warning: Self-awareness alert!)

- "I like it when you show pictures and videos and tell jokes."
- "Sometimes, it is hard for me to understand when you talk too fast."
- "I would like to do more activities where we work with partners and listen to music."
- "I do not like listening to the teacher for a long time without a break."

You will probably get some constructive (and even negative) feedback, and that's OK! Just be aware that your first reaction to criticism may be defensiveness, which is completely natural. Remind yourself of the importance of the work you do, and remember that this exercise will improve outcomes for everyone in your class, including you. Your students receive feedback all day long; it can be very empowering to give them the opportunity to share their input. Exit tickets are just one fun, fast, and enlightening way to solicit feedback.

Once we have student feedback, we can tailor our instruction around what works for students. This simple activity, easily implemented in classrooms or online, helps our students to feel valued, included, and empowered.

Personal Reflection

In what ways do you solicit feedback from your students? How often do you solicit feedback from students?

Developing Interests and Sense of Purpose

"Purpose is the number one, long-term motivator in life."

—William Damon, Professor of Education
Stanford University (Flanagan 2017)

Developing interests gives students the opportunity to express themselves and discover their likes and dislikes. It also helps them to build self-esteem and the satisfaction of developing/progressing with something over time. This process is an integral part of human development. In doing so, we learn to make plans, take directions or instruction, set goals, work through obstacles, and improve our skills. Developing interests is a great start. Building on that, you can ask yourself, *Am I spending my time on things that are important to me?* This question, along with others we share below, are designed to help you and your students in identifying a sense of purpose.

A few things to note about purpose:

- Purpose is not an idea; it is an experience.
- Guiding others to articulate and develop a sense of purpose is enhanced when we have done it ourselves first.
- Purpose tends to become clearer over time.
- Searching for or identifying purpose is a normal and natural part of growing up.
- Being clear about our purpose is a practice that's ongoing and sustained over time, not something we ask ourselves once a year in preparation for the new year.
- People with a sense of purpose tend to live longer, healthier, and happier lives.
- There's no such thing as a purpose that is too big or too small.

Having a sense of purpose is less common among teens (which makes sense given this discovery process is part of being a teen). Not surprisingly, adolescents are more often lectured to than queried about their futures. While we cannot identify purpose for our students or write scripts for their lives, we can:

- Invite students to self-reflect.
- Help students see that they have multiple roles in life (home and family, education and career, community and service, hobbies and recreation, etc.).
- Help young people break down their purpose into achievable goals, and help them take action to achieve those goals.
- Talk to students about what you find meaningful in your career and in your own life. Share with them about the setbacks you have experienced and how you have prevailed.
- Be clear that what they do matters and that what they do has an impact on others for better or worse (Whitlock n.d.).

Personal Reflection

Reflect on purpose in your own life with these questions:

1. What's important to you in your life?

2. What's important to you about being an educator?

3. How do you want to be remembered as an educator?

4. What is the most rewarding thing you have ever done for someone else? Why was it rewarding?

5. If you had all the time in the world to volunteer, who would you volunteer for?

6. What issues do you hold close to your heart?

7. What do you most enjoy spending your time doing?

Spotlight

I have been teaching for 23 years, and 2021 is a new kind of tired. Now, just because it's different doesn't necessarily make it a bad thing. For me, it just means that I need to make adjustments to make sure that my students can be successful. Right now, that looks like them feeling connected to each other and to me. That means adjusting my expectations as well as my instruction. I have to meet them where they are, not where they are "supposed" to be. I remind myself of what I can and cannot control. I cannot control the wind, but I can adjust my sails.

—Sonya Taylor
First Grade Teacher
Jane Adams School
Melrose Park, Illinois

Chapter Summary

Emotion and cognition are connected. When we are able to understand and manage our emotions, it frees us up to engage in more cognitively demanding tasks, such as learning. When it comes to teaching self-awareness skills to students, it is important that we model them ourselves. Self-awareness is important to both a student's academic success as well as their human development. While there are plenty of "behind the scenes" moments for your students to develop self-awareness skills, we encourage you to be clear and explicit with them about the value of self-awareness, offering real-world examples and connections.

Discussion Questions

1. What are your biggest takeaways from this chapter?

2. How can you apply the knowledge you have gained from this chapter?

3. What aspects of self-awareness are you interested in learning more about?

Chapter 2: Self-Management

What Is Self-Management?

Have you ever felt completely overcome by your emotions? Maybe you lost your cool during an argument or sent a text when you were angry. Well, if you have, you're certainly not alone. Everyone at one time or another has felt this way and could benefit from self-management skills.

CASEL defines *self-management* as "the abilities to manage one's emotions, thoughts, and behaviors effectively in different situations and to achieve goals and aspirations." This includes the capacities to delay gratification, manage stress, and feel motivation and agency to accomplish personal and collective goals. One who exhibits self-management can:

- manage his or her emotions
- identify and use stress-management strategies
- exhibit self-discipline and self-motivation
- set personal and collective goals
- use planning and organizational skills
- show the courage to take initiative
- demonstrate personal and collective agency

Why Is Self-Management Important?

When we effectively manage our emotions and cope with stress, our overall sense of well-being improves. We also become better at setting personal and professional goals for ourselves. For students, learning self-management skills is extremely empowering because it allows them the opportunity to develop their abilities to manage their own behaviors. Oftentimes, young children (and even some adults) feel they are powerless over their emotional reactions. When self-management skills are in place, students have heightened senses of personal agency. This reflects externally as being more organized, motivated, and invested in their personal and academic lives.

Our emotions are directly related to our behavior. Students are reprimanded when they express negative behaviors, but beneath every behavior is a need. When we meet that need rather than focus on the behavior, we begin to address the cause and not just the symptom. Classroom management practices that punish students for expressing themselves will not solve the problem; in fact, it wastes valuable instructional time. To be clear, SEL is not a classroom-management framework. However, when students learn how to better manage themselves, educators and students can both focus their energies on the all-important work of teaching and learning. This shift from teacher-centered classroom management to student-centered self-management promotes a classroom culture that focuses on the needs, abilities, interests, and learning styles of its students.

Managing Emotions

In the previous chapter on self-awareness, we learned that emotions are important messages, each containing vital pieces of information. The main purposes of emotions are to:

- take action
- survive
- avoid danger
- make decisions
- understand others (Cherry 2020)

Learning how to identify our emotions sets the stage for the next important skill: managing our emotions. Regulating emotions does not mean eliminating emotions—it means using them to help us gain a better understanding of ourselves. We cannot choose our emotions, but we can choose how we respond to them.

Here's an example: someone cuts you off in traffic. You immediately experience anger. Your heart might start beating quickly, and you might feel the urge to lash out. Maybe you yell or honk the horn. In that moment, believe it or not, you have a *choice*. You have the option to *react* or to *respond*. If you react to your emotions, you give yourself very little time and act on impulse. But if you respond, you can take a moment to recognize the signs of your anger (e.g., heart rate, raised voice), label your emotion (I'm angry), and then decide how you want to respond moving forward.

Reacting when we are experiencing strong emotions (such as anger, sadness, disgust, frustration) leaves no time to fairly weigh potential outcomes and often leads to unwanted consequences. As a result, it is rare that we make our lives easier when we make decisions at the height of our emotional state. Being able to observe our emotions—even when they feel overwhelmingly powerful—creates a space in which we can more adequately weigh the consequences of our actions.

Identifying Stress

What do we know about stress? Once upon a time, stress helped human beings avoid being eaten by wooly mammoths. However, *chronic* and *high* levels of stress can be downright toxic to our minds and bodies. And while the physical and biological effects of stress (dilated pupils, increased heartbeat) prepare us to engage in "fight or flight," they render us far less receptive to learning. Young people are affected when the adults in their lives are stressed out. This is one of the reasons why SEL starts with adults. Once we identify our own personal stressors, we will be more capable in supporting students to acknowledge and explore their own stress levels.

 # Personal Reflection

What stresses you out? How do you feel or act when you are stressed? How does it impact you when someone around you is stressed out?

Kinds of Stress

Not all stress is created equal. What contributes to stress can vary greatly from person to person and differs according to various social and economic circumstances. Children who grow up experiencing significant adversity or trauma experience toxic levels of stress. Growing up in a household or community where we experience unpredictability and high levels of emotional or physical threat will very likely alter our stress response (Perry and Winfrey 2021). Some stress is "good stress" because it is associated with goal achievement, like finishing a project or college applications. However, this is very different from the chronic and continual stress ("bad stress") of having the electricity shut off, the uncertainty of living paycheck to paycheck, experiencing food insecurity, or growing up with unstable parenting. As a result, students who belong to marginalized and historically underserved populations experience more "bad stress" more frequently. The toxic stress of racism also contributes to adverse mental and physical health effects in people of color (Comas-Diaz et al. 2019). Racism yields racial inequities and disparities in every sector of private and public life, including but not limited to politics, health care, criminal justice, education, income, employment, and home ownership. CASEL identifies practicing anti-racism as a self-management skill. At the start of the 2021–22 school year, districts and educators all across the country engaged in the all-important work of anti-racist professional development. An *anti-racist educator* actively works to dismantle the structures, policies, institutions, and systems that create barriers and perpetuate race-based inequities for people of color (Simmons 2019). SEL is most effective when stakeholders understand the effects that systemic racism has on their students of color, their families, and their communities.

Educators and Stress

Your health and well-being are a priority. However, educator "self-care" is not meant to be one more thing a teacher feels like they have to do. Ironically, feeling like we have to do something just adds to our stress. Educators deserve school and district-wide policies that support well-being. Educators and school staff are some of the most selfless people on Earth, but we are here to remind you to put on your oxygen mask first (in other words, learn stress-management skills) before you assist others. You are too important to let your needs take a backseat. And you are not able to be as effective in your role when you feel drained. When we have nothing left to give, what do we have to offer? "Studies have shown that teachers with stronger social and emotional competencies are less likely to report burnout, demonstrate higher levels of patience and empathy, and have more positive relationships with students, contributing to their academic, social and emotional development" (Schlund, Jagers, and Schlinger 2020). It's easy to get swept up in the idea that we need to be "productive" all the time. We're going to let you in on a little secret, so lean in. Sometimes, the most productive thing we can do is rest.

Managing Stress

There is not a one-size-fits-all approach when it comes to managing stress. Everyone is different, so it is important to find stress-management techniques that work best for us. Young people learn how to take care of themselves when they see us effectively take care of ourselves. Stressful moments are inevitable. Rather than trying to hide it, students can benefit when they see adults and peers effectively manage stress and self-regulate. When educators have strong self-management skills, they serve as role models for their students.

Stress Management Personal Inventory

When we are stressed, we often forget some of the most basic ways to take care of ourselves. Read the statements in the chart, and put a check mark in the column that best describes how you respond. Are you attending to some of these basic ways of reducing stress?

	This is not happening.	I'm on my way but could use a little help.	I'm pretty good at this.	Nailing it!
I'm eating well. I eat foods that nourish my body.				
I exercise or move my body during the day.				
My quality of sleep is good. (I do not have trouble falling asleep or staying asleep.)				
I drink enough water during the day.				
I treat myself like I would a good friend or family member.				
I'm aware of my breathing during the day.				

Personal Reflection

How are you prioritizing your own health and wellness? Where would you like to improve?

Motivation

Another aspect of self-management is *motivation*. For this section, we'd like to take you on a little trip back in time.

 ## Storytime

I am a first-year teacher, working with a group of eighth-graders to prepare them for the upcoming Constitution test. I have one student, Alex, who simply will not complete the study guide. So, I incentivize (bribe) him with his favorite candy bar. The next day, Alex turns in the completed study guide, and I hand him the candy bar (a real quid pro quo). A few days later, when it is time to take the test, Alex says he does not want to take the exam. When I ask him why, he replies, "If a study guide is worth one bar, the test must be worth about three bars, but I'm definitely not doing it for free."

What happened here?

By providing an external incentive, I assigned a value (specifically, one candy bar) to the task at hand. I drained all the potential for Alex to self-motivate. By trying to bribe him, I inadvertently sent the message that this work was drudgery and the only way to slog through it was to be compensated.

We know from experience that external rewards work in the short term. Whether it is candy, pizza, or bonus bucks, they work like a charm. Why? For the same reason people like to go to casinos. DOPAMINE!

That's right, Alex's brain got a little burst of the feel-good chemical dopamine. But constantly providing incentives in the form of external rewards does not work in the long term. I made the mistake of trying to coax effort out of Alex. Alex did not care about the test because it had not been made relevant for him. In hindsight, I should have validated Alex's negotiation skills; alas, I did not. I also failed to provide Alex with a rationale for what he was doing. I did not take the time to make a connection between the content and his real life. Unfortunately, some behavior-management programs punish students for lack of motivation to get compliance. The problem is that compliance is mostly effective for routine work. Students are more motivated when they can assign meaning to something. I denied Alex what researcher Daniel Pink (2011) calls the three ingredients of genuine motivation: *autonomy*, *mastery*, and *purpose*.

- *Autonomy* is the urge to direct one's own life. In classrooms, it means students have voice and choice.
- *Mastery* is the desire to get better at something that matters. In classrooms, it means students understand that many failures will occur before mastery is achieved.
- *Purpose* is the yearning to do work in the service of something larger than one's self. In school, this means feeling like an integral part of the classroom and school culture.

Personal Reflection

In your classroom, how are students being provided with autonomy, mastery, and purpose? What does that look like?

Vision Board

One way for students to illustrate what has meaning and to help clarify specific goals is to create vision boards. A vision board is any sort of "board" (paper or digital) to display images that represent whatever you want to do, be, or have in your life. When students create vision boards, it helps them connect with what motivates and inspires them. When they share their vision boards, it helps them to connect with one another. (See Figure 2.1 below.)

Figure 2.1: Sample Vision Board

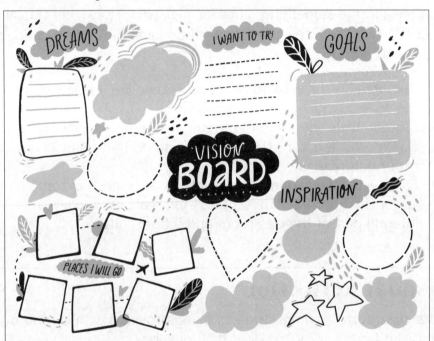

Goal Setting

Goal setting is a powerful strategy that gives students the opportunity to identify something that's important to them while experiencing pride in their accomplishments. The very act of creating a goal takes courage. Think about the last time you set a goal. Was it exciting and a bit nerve-racking?

Part of setting ourselves up for success is setting an appropriate goal. One technique we like to use for goal setting is the SMART framework (Doran 1981).

Let's check out what the SMART acronym stands for.

Acronym	Stands for...	In other words...
S	Specific	Is the goal clear and precise?
M	Measurable	How will I know I've accomplished it?
A	Attainable	Is it a stretch but not impossible?
R	Relevant	What is important to me about the goal?
T	Time bound	Does it have a "by when" date?

Developing a SMART goal is all about relevance and helping students discover what is important to them about the goal.

The second goal-setting strategy is PACT, which is the acronym for **P**urposeful, **A**ctionable, **C**ontinuous, and **T**rackable. PACT goals focus on output whereas SMART goals focus on outcome. The PACT technique works especially well for long-term, ambitious goals because they are focused on continuous growth. This strategy is usually more useful for goals that require on-going effort like learning to code or play the violin. When writing PACT goals, there are four things to consider.

Acronym	Stands for...	In other words...
P	Purposeful	It speaks to your values and fuels your ambitions and actions.
A	Actionable	You are making effort to change things within your reach and control.
C	Continuous	The action you take is sustainable and can be consistently performed.
T	Trackable	Your effort and progress can be tracked.

An example of a SMART Goal is: "I'm going to run a 5K by March 27th" whereas a PACT goal is: "I'm going to run every day of this year."

Oftentimes, we can accidentally project what *we* think should be important for our students or what *we* think their goals should be.

Having goal setting be a student-led experience will get them more engaged in the process. Sharing a goal you have set is also a great way to build connections with students and get them excited about setting their own.

 # Spotlight

Imagine you have 27 senior high school students and you have been tasked with teaching them *Hamlet* or *Beowulf*. Seems like the perfect storm of disinterest, right? So, how did I get these students to engage in these great works? How did I show them that the skills we use to investigate great works of literature are applicable to, well, everything?

I gave them choice and an outlet for their creativity and curiosity. I did so by implementing a 20 percent project.

What is a 20 percent project?

Simply put, it is a semester-long project that requires students to pick a goal, write a contract, and build a project that will allow them to showcase the skills they learned throughout the semester. Students work on the project one day a week, or 20 percent of the school week. The best part is that when a student knows they have time to work exclusively on their passions, build something completely on their own, and work on it at their own pace, they are a heck of a lot more engaged throughout the week. They feel empowered to direct their own learning and emboldened to make connections between the literature we are analyzing and the content they are shaping for themselves. I want my classroom to be a place where students have voice, choice, and agency. Instead of me telling them what to do, I invite them to show me what they can do.

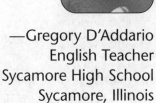

—Gregory D'Addario
English Teacher
Sycamore High School
Sycamore, Illinois

SEL in Action

Setting goals is just the start. Remind students, once you have set a goal, there will be ups and downs and plot twists along the way. Here are five tips to help your students overcome these inevitable obstacles:

Obstacle:	Tip:	For example:
Goals feel overwhelming.	**Tip:** Take small steps. If we make our steps too big, we are not likely to do them. Break your goal down into smaller, more bite-size pieces. This gives us the greatest chance to experience success. This leads to momentum and, you guessed it, more steps. Taking small steps consistently is much more likely to work compared to over-promising a large accomplishment at one time (which is often unrealistic).	**For example:** If a student sets a goal to read a book during the semester, have them start small, perhaps reading a couple of pages at a time and ultimately building up to one chapter per sitting.
It takes too long to accomplish the goal.	**Tip:** Celebrate accomplishments along the way. Celebrating is not reserved only for when you achieve the goal. Particularly when we are doing something new, each step we take requires a lot of energy and effort. Give your students the opportunity to celebrate their successes along the way—it is more engaging and motivating when we pause to celebrate the small wins alongside the big ones.	**For example:** Using visual representations to show how close they are getting to their goals can help mark the small wins. Use journals to keep track of their accomplishments and reflect on the challenges they have overcome.

Obstacle:	Tip:	For example:
It is hard to stay committed to the goal.	Students will inevitably get "stuck" at some point in trying to reach their goals. Call in support. The first step to calling in support is sharing your goal with someone—because it becomes a declaration: "I'm going to do this!" Pair your students with a check-in buddy (account-a-bili-buddy!) so they can support each other.	Here are a few questions teachers can ask students to identify the support they need: Who might be able to help you? How can I help you? What resources are available that would help you reach your goal? What's the most challenging part right now? Where do you feel you're getting stuck? What would the smallest next step be?
Obstacle: It is hard to remember the goal.	Tip: Make the goal visible. Having students display their goals somewhere they can see them helps keep the goals "in front" of them. There is wisdom in the old saying "out of sight, out of mind."	For example: Here are ways to keep the goal visible: Create a goal "garden" for your entire classroom to display their goals. Have students display their goals on their desks. Have students post their goals at home (on the refrigerator, by their beds, desks, or bathroom mirrors).
Obstacle: It feels like no progress is being made.	Tip: Track your progress. We all love seeing progress! Have students track their accomplishments along the way.	For example: Use something simple like a "goal thermometer" to continually monitor progress. Older students can write letters from their future selves, congratulating themselves on their accomplishments as if they have already happened and explaining how satisfied they feel.

Personal and Collective Agency

 "Everything can be taken from a man but one thing: The last of the human freedoms—to choose one's attitude in any given set of circumstances, to choose one's own way."

—Viktor E. Frankl (1946)

Personal agency means we recognize we are in control of whether we *react* or *respond*. *Agency* does not imply that someone is good or bad— it simply refers to the degree of perceived control someone has in their life. What we are most interested in is how to foster a strong sense of personal agency so that students and educators alike see themselves in the driver's seat of their own lives. In doing so, we are more engaged and make better decisions.

When someone has personal agency, they are more likely to partake in *collective agency*, to come and act together for a specific cause or reason. Collective agency is important because it is the ability to look beyond one's self to see a larger collective context, like your class, school, neighborhood, city, state, or country.

Chapter Summary

Educators have long recognized the importance of self-management skills. Effectively managing emotions takes place when we understand that while we cannot choose our emotions, we can choose how we respond to them. In terms of stress, finding the best management strategies may take some experimenting and require some practice. The more we practice, the more it becomes automatic. The main thing is, we keep looking for the tools that will help manage life's inevitable ups and downs in a healthy way.

Discussion Questions

1. What are your biggest takeaways from this chapter?

2. How can you apply the knowledge you have gained from this chapter?

3. What aspects of self-management are you interested in learning more about?

Chapter 3: Social Awareness

What Is Social Awareness?

Looking at what has been covered so far, you have probably noticed that all five SEL competencies are interrelated. GO YOU! As you develop the capacity to better recognize and understand the cause of your own emotions (*self-awareness*), you will find it easier to appreciate the perspectives and feelings of others (*social awareness*).

CASEL defines *social awareness* as "the ability to understand the perspectives of and empathize with others, including those from diverse backgrounds, cultures, and contexts. This includes the capacities to feel compassion for others, understand broader historical and social norms for behavior in different settings, and recognize family, school, and community resources and support." One who is socially aware can:

- see others' perspectives
- recognize strengths in others
- demonstrate empathy and compassion
- show concern for the feelings of others
- understand and express gratitude
- identify diverse social norms, including unjust ones
- recognize situational demands and opportunities
- understand the influences of systems on behavior

Why Is Social Awareness Important?

Social and emotional learning is, of course, social, meaning interacting with individuals, groups, and society. Society is complex. For stakeholders in education, being socially aware includes acknowledging the persistent inequities in education that undermine opportunities for students to learn in deep and meaningful ways. These inequities may be rooted in race/ethnicity, sexual orientation, social class, home language, etc. (CASEL 2021). For example, "LGBTQ students report the greatest levels of anxiety and depression. LGBTQ youth in the United States experience greater rates of bullying and lower academic achievement than their non LGBTQ peers." (Brackett 2019, 191). While SEL might not be the antidote to all societal issues, it can be a part of the solution. SEL is about connection, and empathy can be a powerful tool to connect individuals across culture, race, or language.

Empathy

A great way to build connections with others is through empathy. *Empathy* is from the Greek *empatheia* (from *em–* 'in' + *pathos* 'feeling'), and it is a term that is gaining a lot of popularity—not just in education but also in medical fields, sports, and even sales. The concept of empathy is interpreted in many ways. For the purposes of SEL, we define *empathy* as the ability to understand and respond to the feelings of others (Ashoka United States, n.d.). It means being curious about understanding another's perspective and looking beyond your own point of view. While it is not possible to perfectly inhabit another person's experience, there is great value in imagining what others may be thinking or experiencing. Ask yourself how you would feel in their shoes. Once someone can do that, they can move from *feeling* empathy to *acting* on it. Taking action from a place of empathy is what helps us to build and maintain connections with students, parents, coworkers—basically, everyone.

It is worth noting that empathizing with someone and seeing their point of view does not necessarily mean you agree with them. Contrary to what we may see on social media, we do have the capacity to respectfully disagree with others. Studies indicate that when young people have empathy, they display

- higher academic achievement,
- better communication skills,
- lower likelihood of bullying,
- fewer aggressive behaviors and emotional disorders, and
- more positive relationships (Jones et al. n.d.).

 ## Personal Reflection

In a conversation, do you wonder about the other person's perspective? Do you hear what the other person is saying, or are you more concerned with them simply hearing you?

Empathy in Action

We know teachers want tangible support to use in their classrooms. That's why we, with the help of an amazing veteran teacher (Michelle Delarosa), created a tool to help us build that empathy muscle. **CALM** is a simple framework that supports educators in taking a more empathetic approach by prioritizing *responding* over *reacting*.

CALM stands for **C**heck yourself; **A**sk yourself; **L**isten; **M**anage your actions.

Scenario	What Is Happening?
Student misbehaves	Student is expressing a need; there may not be a negative intention toward you or behind the behavior. It may be a call for connection.
Get **CALM**	
Check yourself: Am I *reacting*?	How am I feeling? How is my body reacting to this situation? Am I taking this personally?
Ask yourself: Check for bias, judgements, underlying beliefs.	What assumptions am I making about this student right now? What do I know about the student or the situation? Is this behavior disruptive, or can I continue instruction?
Listen: Gather evidence by checking in and checking on the student from a place of curiosity.	What's going on? How are you feeling? What do you need right now? Is there anything you want me to know?
Manage your actions: *Respond* rather than *react*.	When we have more information, we are better equipped to address the situation at its root and act from a place of empathy.

Let's look at a real-life classroom scenario that took place with one of our students. Remember, it is normal to have thoughts similar to those in the left-hand column.

Scenario: A visibly tired student keeps putting their head down and dozing off in class.

WITHOUT CALM Reactive	WITH CALM Responsive
This impacts me. • Am I that boring? • How disrespectful! • I cannot believe they are sleeping during a lesson that I worked so hard on.	**C**heck Yourself • It is not about me. • My role is to help them, not judge them. • What story am I telling myself about this student? • Am I taking this behavior personally?
I make an assumption. • Do I need to nip this in the bud so the class knows this is not acceptable behavior? • This student is breaking rules on purpose.	**A**sk Yourself • What do I actually know about this student? • How could I find out more?
I take an authoritarian action. • I need to issue a consequence and move on. • This behavior deserves a punishment.	**L**isten • I notice you seem tired. What's going on? • Is there anything you want me to know?
I want a quick solution. • I write them up. • I call them out and reprimand them publicly.	**M**anage your Actions • Now that I have more perspective, I can decide when and how to help the student.

To continue the story, after asking the student why they were tired, we found out that they were up late helping one of their parents at work. This new information helped elicit a more empathetic response and strengthened our relationship. Huzzah!

SEL in Action

Ready to give it a shot? Consider the scenario, and imagine how you may have *reacted* in the past (which may not have been all that empathetic—no shame). Then, apply CALM to see how you could *respond* instead.

Scenario: A student has been missing school and not turning in their homework.

WITHOUT CALM Reactive	WITH CALM Responsive
This impacts me:	**C**heck yourself:
I make an assumption:	**A**sk yourself:
I take an authoritarian action:	**L**isten:
I want a quick solution:	**M**anage your actions:

What do you notice about the two columns? How could you remind yourself to stay CALM?

Storytime

One morning, one of my high school students walked into my classroom and said, "Miss, you got a pimple." Now, you can imagine what my initial reaction was to having this information broadcast for my entire class to hear. I felt embarrassed and, quite frankly, a little upset. I wanted to *react* to this comment immediately. My first thought was that she was intentionally trying to disrespect me. Fortunately, we had recently had a professional development session where we focused on *responding* instead of *reacting*. So, I took a moment and instead of accusing her of what I thought her intention was, I decided to get curious.

"Why are you telling me this?" I inquired.

"Because, Miss, if you go to the bathroom, you can take care of it, and I'll watch the class for you."

She said this as if it were the most obvious reason in the world. She was being sincere and never intended to harm me by stating the fact (I mean, I did have a pimple). She was simply looking out for me. If I had not paused and gotten curious, I could have potentially damaged our relationship.

Ways to Teach Empathy

Research shows that we all vary in how much we experience empathy. It is important to remember that having and demonstrating empathy can vary from situation to situation. This skill set can also develop at different speeds.

Model Empathy

It is important that students understand what empathy looks and sounds like. It is especially helpful to verbally articulate your thought process when modeling empathy. For example, the next time you are frustrated, you can share how you are feeling with your students and discuss ways you can deal with your frustration.

Explicitly Teach Empathy

Provide explicit instruction about what empathy is and how it benefits students. Discuss the importance of having empathy for individuals who are different from you. The more real-world connections students can make, the more motivated they will be to try it themselves. Ask students to reflect on experiences where they reacted empathetically to situations or may have received empathetic responses.

Praise Empathy

Validate and praise students who demonstrate empathy! Make the praise specific and meaningful. For example, a student checks in on a student who is not feeling well. Call it out! "You saw Jordan wasn't feeling well, and you asked if there was anything you could do to help him out today. That was very empathetic of you." Or a student finishes his assignment early and turns to help his tablemate. Provide praise: "You saw Adrian was struggling, and you offered to help him. That was very empathetic of you."

The more students experience empathy, the more likely they are to offer it to others. Look for opportunities throughout the day to model, teach, and praise when students are displaying empathy. Call it out! When students see empathy publicly recognized, they will start to look for ways to be empathetic themselves.

Use Reflection to Build Empathy

> "We do not learn from experience... we learn from reflection on experience."
>
> —John Dewey (1933, 78)

We need to purposefully reflect on our responses to build empathy. The reflection questions in this book are designed for this purpose. Reflecting on common scenarios, like the two previously mentioned, is an important part of the process of becoming more self- and socially aware. Reflection enhances learning because it encourages *metacognition*, which is a fancy word for "thinking about our thinking." Metacognition is an essential skill for learner success because it helps students reflect on who they are, what they know, and why it is important. Self-reflection is integral in developing all five SEL competencies and, in particular, to learning empathy. As we like to say, having students engage in an activity without giving them time to reflect on their learning is like working on a term paper all night and slamming your laptop closed without clicking "save."

Calling In versus Calling Out

Developing social awareness and empathy skills means being able to engage with people who have different perspectives than we do. When we "call someone out," we are usually assuming the worst and shaming the other person for thinking or acting a certain way. While shame can be an immediate motivator, it is not an authentic one. Shame motivates out of a place of fear. Validation motivates from a place of love and understanding. We have missed out on any valuable learning! This leads to little or no possibility of having an open conversation. Now, if this sounds at all familiar to you, you are not alone. When we are not happy with someone, we might be tempted to "call them out" over text, social media, or in a heated exchange face-to-face. While it may feel good for a moment, it does not often lead to any resolution or satisfying outcome.

"Some people you can work with and some people you can work around. But the thing that I want to emphasize is that the calling-in practice means you always keep a seat at the table for them if they come back."

—Loretta J. Ross (Bennett 2020)

Scenario: We hear a teacher repeatedly refer to several students as the "bad kids" in class.

Call Out: We could "call out" this teacher by telling other coworkers or talking behind the teacher's back. Would this improve outcomes for students? Would this contribute to a positive climate in our school? How does it feel to be the teacher on the giving or receiving end?

So, let's look at an alternative. What if we "called people in?" "Calling in" involves conversation, compassion, and context. It involves taking a breath before commenting, or firing off an email or text. It is still creating accountability but without casting someone into exile. In doing so, we can remain curious and create an opportunity for an open conversation. How could we "call in" this teacher?

Call In: Have a one-on-one conversation with the teacher. Maybe ask some clarifying questions to help them see that while student *behaviors* might be negative, students are not *bad*. We could even see what strengths this teacher currently has and consider how to help harness those strengths to benefit students. Now, when we ask ourselves, "Could this improve outcomes for our students? Would this contribute to a positive climate in our school?" we can confidently answer "Yes!"

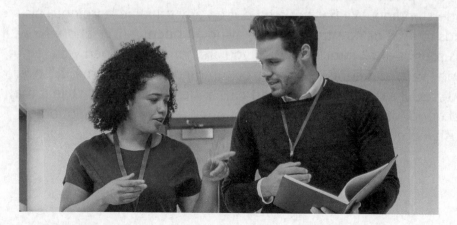

Systemic Racism

 "Not everything that is faced can be changed, but nothing can be changed until it is faced."

—James Baldwin (n.d.)

To meet the needs of all our students and adults, we need to acknowledge the root causes of inequity. You have probably heard the term *systemic racism* in many contexts recently. *Systemic racism* refers to the systems in place that create and maintain racial inequality in nearly every facet of life for people of color (Yancey-Bragg 2020). It is called *systemic* racism because it can be found in the policies and practices at institutions like banks, schools, companies, government agencies, and law enforcement. Systemic racism is hard for people to grasp because it is all around us and does not have a face. As a result, it can be very difficult for some people to see all the ways in which systemic racism impacts the daily lives of people in our country. Here's a parable to illustrate that sometimes something obvious can be hard to see and talk about.

> Two young fish are swimming along and they happen upon an older fish swimming the other way. The older fish nods at them and says, "Morning, boys. How's the water?" And the two young fish swim on for a bit, and then eventually one of them looks over at the other and goes, "What the heck is water?" (Wallace 2005).

One example of how systemic racism has impacted and continues to impact schools is redlining. *Redlining* is a discriminatory practice that puts services (financial and otherwise) out of reach for residents of certain areas based on race or ethnicity. It can be seen in the systematic denial of mortgages, insurance, loans, and other financial services based on location rather than on an individual's qualifications. The term *redlining* was coined because banks would use red ink on a map to outline parts of cities they deemed as having an undesirable population to lend to (most notably minority neighborhoods). Loans in these neighborhoods were unavailable or very expensive, making it more difficult for low-income minorities to buy homes. Consequently, many communities missed out on decades of homeownership, which is one of the top contributors to accumulating wealth in the United States. The inability to reap these benefits has also contributed to the country's persistent racial wealth gap. While the Fair Housing Act of 1968 put an end to legally sanctioned redlining policies, new forms of redlining show up as predatory lending (especially during the 2008 housing crisis) and within institutions outside the mortgage industry.

Redlining is just one example of how a racist policy can impact our students of color. These racial inequities and disparities appear in every sector of private and public life, including education, politics, health care, criminal justice, income, employment, and home ownership. At the end of the day, SEL is most effective when stakeholders understand the effects that systemic racism has on their students of color, their families, and their communities. Policies impact all our lives for better or for worse. Understanding the influences of organizations and systems on behavior is an essential part of social awareness.

 Personal Reflection

How have institutional policies (e.g., federal, education) impacted your own life in positive ways? How have they impacted your life in negative ways?

Recognizing Support and Resources

You, me, and the most successful people you know all have 1,440 minutes in a day. So, the question becomes, how do you use your 1,440 minutes? It's funny—in the United States in particular, we have this notion that we are supposed to do everything by ourselves (rugged individualism!). However, one thing that successful people have in common is they have very good support systems. Just look at anyone that you admire or consider very successful. Do you notice the ways in which they have called in support and resources? It is highly unlikely they got to where they are by doing everything by themselves.

When we let others support us, we can reach our goals faster and with more ease. Creating support systems and recognizing resources can look many different ways. It could be anything from finding a therapist to phoning a friend for help. Most importantly, start noticing when you can reach out rather than trying to do everything yourself.

The bonus of calling in support is that the other person gets the feel-good perks from helping. Don't you enjoy when you get to lend a helping hand? You wouldn't want to deny someone else that feeling. You can let them help you!

The 5 Ws of Support

Most people are pretty good at giving support. We are not quite as comfortable receiving it. Use the 5 *Ws* (*Who*, *What*, *Where*, *When*, and *Why*; see Figure 3.1) to help yourself identify how to find the support and help you need.

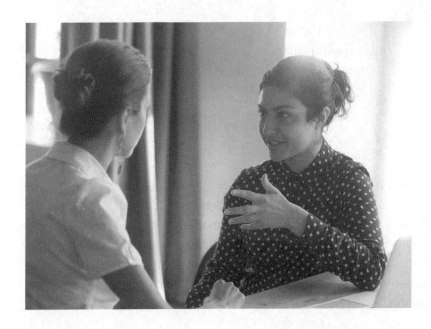

Figure 3.1: The 5 Ws of Support

	Ask	**Consider**
Who	Who might support me with this?	friends, family, colleagues, classmates, mentors, advisors, or people who offer conventional forms of support, such as mental-health professionals
What	What resources are available at school?	a colleague, your site administrator, a school counselor, or a health-care professional
Where	Where else could I look for support?	community office, health department, or outside organization that can point you in the right direction
When	When am I going to take action?	a plan or structure that might be useful, such as setting calendar reminders or asking a friend to check in
Why?	Why am I doing this?	the benefits of taking action and why it's important to you

Gratitude: It Is Not Just for Thanksgiving

"The little things? The little moments? They aren't little. Saying thank you, holding the door for someone, these little moments can change the tone of your whole day."

—Jon Kabat-Zinn (1994)

Gratitude is a practice. It literally makes you feel happier. And guess what? Your brain just *loves* it. It gobbles gratitude right up. Many studies over the past decade have found that people who consciously identify and focus on the good things tend to be happier, feel less pain and stress, suffer insomnia less, have stronger immune systems, experience healthier relationships, and do better academically and professionally (*Psychology Today* Staff n.d.). Yes, please, sign us up!

SEL in Action

If practicing gratitude is like working a muscle, how are you strengthening yours? Here are a few ways to practice gratitude yourself and how you can help your students exercise gratitude as well.

Gratitude Exercises for You	Gratitude Exercises for Students
Keep a gratitude journal. Journal, voice-record, or in some other way take note of the big and little joys of daily life. Include ordinary events, people, or something simple you enjoyed.	**Record gratitude daily.** A daily exit ticket or a turn-and-talk with a friend will remind students to take a moment to be grateful.
Share your gratitude with others. Write thank-you notes to others, or simply let them know what you appreciate about them.	**Post office.** Have a center filled with paper, crayons, markers, stickers, and more, and encourage students to leave notes of gratitude for their friends. **Hint:** You can also leave notes for your students!
Use visuals. Think about people who have inspired you. What about them was most significant? Have their pictures (or quotes) posted somewhere you can see them easily and regularly.	**Mementos.** Encourage students to bring in photos or other trinkets that remind them of the people they care about. Students can write about what they brought or share in small groups. Students should also have the option *not* to share.
Be mindful of your language. Start to notice the words you're using to describe daily events and others. Is there mention of what you appreciate, what you're grateful for, what is possible, or where there is benefit?	**Turn *No* into *Yes*.** So often, students only hear what they *cannot* do. Use language that gives them positive options, and encourage them to do the same. For example, instead of saying, "You cannot change your seat," try saying, "You can switch seats after the activity is finished."

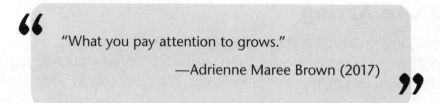

"What you pay attention to grows."

—Adrienne Maree Brown (2017)

Recognizing Situational Demands

Different situations call for different behaviors and language choices. The way you talk in a job interview is likely to be different than how you talk with your friends. Our students are faced with a myriad of situational demands. The goal is to support students in navigating each of the situations so they can be successful. We best support students when we validate who they are culturally and linguistically.

To be clear, supporting a student to express themselves in standard English in a job interview should in no way negate or invalidate the value of the language they use with their friends or how they interact with their families at home. All languages are valid. The best way to support our students is to see them through an asset-based lens so we can affirm the values, cultures, languages, and lived experiences of all students.

 ## Personal Reflection

Does your use of language change in different situations? If so, how, and why?

Chapter Summary

Social awareness can foster equitable outcomes that extend beyond any individual success and influence communities and society. When we engage students in learning about their own and others' identities, cultures, and backgrounds, we are creating a sense of connectedness. This sense of belonging and trust is the foundation upon which we can engage students in broader conversations around social and historical issues of equity. Additionally, when we assist students in developing their capacities to seek help, practice gratitude, and demonstrate empathy, they are better equipped for professional and personal success. Social awareness skills help students navigate the world with more ease.

Discussion Questions

1. What are your biggest takeaways from this chapter?

2. How can you apply the knowledge you have gained from this chapter?

3. What aspects of social awareness are you interested in learning more about?

Chapter 4: Relationship Skills

What Are Relationship Skills?

Positive relationships are the soil in which SEL skills grow. We are social creatures. We are meant to live in communities where we are connected to others. Relationships provide that connection. When we as adults experience successful relationships and a sense of connectedness and belonging, we feel better. The same is true for our students.

CASEL defines *relationship skills* as "the abilities to establish and maintain healthy and supportive relationships and to effectively navigate settings with diverse individuals and groups." This includes the capacities to communicate clearly, listen actively, cooperate, work collaboratively to problem-solve and negotiate conflict constructively, navigate settings with differing social and cultural demands and opportunities, provide leadership, and seek or offer help when needed. One who exhibits positive relationship skills can:

- communicate effectively
- develop positive relationships
- demonstrate cultural competency
- practice teamwork and collaborative problem-solving
- resolve conflicts constructively
- resist negative social pressure
- show leadership in groups
- seek or offer support and help when needed
- stand up for the rights of others

Why Are Relationship Skills Important?

At the most fundamental level, we are designed for human connection. Relationships in schools—with stakeholders and peers—have the potential to have long-lasting impacts on students. Specifically, teacher-student relationships can promote school success in the following ways:

- strengthen academic achievement
- reduce chronic absenteeism
- promote self-motivation
- strengthen self-regulation
- improve goal-making skills

Strong connections with students create positive classroom environments where teachers can spend more time and energy on teaching rather than managing classroom behavior. When students have positive interactions with adults, they exhibit fewer behavior issues. Students who have meaningful connections with their teachers are also more likely to form similar relationships in the future (Waterford.org 2019).

Personal Reflection

Think of someone who helped you become the person you are today. How did you feel being around them? How did they treat you?

Developing Positive Relationships

Relationships are a two-way street. It is easy for educators to feel that sharing about themselves will diminish their authority and control. The truth is, showing vulnerability actually generates more respect from students. Generally, when you open up to students, they tend to take the cue that it is safe to open up to you. Your students want to know you. Think about when you run into a student in the store. They feel like they have spotted you out in the wild (this is especially true of younger students). In their minds, you live in the classroom where you sleep in a Murphy bed that comes out of the wall. You can share small things about yourself and your life that can help foster a sense of connection. It can be something as simple as introducing any pets you have or talking about your favorite hobby. The point is, they want to know who you are as a person.

Keys to Connection Checklist

We can all contribute to the emotional development of young people. However, sometimes we just don't know where to begin. Or maybe we can tell something is not quite right with a student, but we just can't put our finger on what it is. This checklist (Figure 4.1 below) gives you a clear and tangible place to start. We have witnessed firsthand how this list has supported educators in transforming and enhancing the quality of their connections with students. Heck, it can even help increase connecting with your in-laws.

Figure 4.1: Keys to Connection Checklist

☐ accepted	☐ forgiven	☐ respected
☐ acknowledged	☐ heard	☐ safe
☐ admired	☐ helpful	☐ supported
☐ appreciated	☐ important	☐ treated fairly
☐ approved of	☐ included	☐ trusted
☐ believed in	☐ in control	☐ understood
☐ capable	☐ listened to	☐ useful
☐ challenged	☐ loved	☐ validated
☐ competent	☐ needed	☐ valued
☐ confident	☐ noticed	☐ worthy

For example, let's say I am having difficulty with a particular student. Let's call him Junior. I can use this checklist to assess how many ways I am currently connecting to Junior. Does Junior feel accepted by me? Does Junior feel acknowledged by me? And so on. Then, let's say I realized that Junior does *not* feel appreciated by me. I can then use this newfound insight and make an effort to communicate to Junior one or two specific ways that I appreciate him. The power of this process is the inventory we take of our relationships with students. This information can then help guide future decisions and interactions. **Note:** You do not need to "check off" every key on the checklist for every student.

Spotlight

One strategy that was extremely helpful to engage my high school students during remote learning was a *daily check-in question*. These check-in questions ranged from thought-provoking to silly. My students generally did not have their cameras on. One day, the check-in question was "Show me something that brings you joy." After much encouragement from me, one of my students, Damian, finally replied. He wrote in the chat box, "The piano my dad gave me." I enthusiastically proceeded to ask him about his playing. Several minutes went by, and he did not respond. I had just moved on to another student when suddenly, we all heard the first tentative notes of a piano being played. Soon, our whole virtual room was filled with this most exquisite piece of classical music. The entire class was enraptured by Damian's playing. Then, just as quickly as it had begun, the piece ended and Damian turned his microphone off. There was total silence for a beat and then, without cue, every student turned on their mics and cheered and applauded uproariously for our talented Damian. For the rest of the year, the class spoke and connected with Damian about his beautiful piano music. We all learned about and connected to Damian that day. Turns out all we needed to do was ask.

—Karen L. Smith
English Teacher, Lloyde High School
Lawndale, California

SEL in Action

Once you have an inventory of different ways you are connecting to a student, you can take positive steps to build on those connections or to address ones you are missing with a few simple moves. Here are several strategies that promote keys to connection.

Keys to Connection	Strategies
Believed In Students want to feel believed in by their teachers, families, and classmates.	• Provide encouragement. • Facilitate and acknowledge small successes. • Tell them you believe in them and why (e.g., "You can do it. I believe in you. You're stronger than you know.").
In Control Students feel in control when they have choices. Choices also help improve engagement and motivation.	• Engage students as leaders, problem solvers, and decision makers. • Have students vote on what, when, or how they do an activity (e.g., "Do you want to work independently or in groups?")
Respected Students are more likely to respect teachers who they feel respect them. It is a two-way street. (This is especially important in secondary and high school.)	• Utilize policies and practices that are restorative and equitably applied. • Create an inclusive culture that fosters caring relationships. • Avoid power struggles. • Show them respect.
Treated Fairly Students feel they are treated fairly when they understand classroom rules and consequences. When rules and consequences are made clear to students, it helps take the teacher out of the equation so that students do not feel judged.	• Include students in creating the classroom rules and consequences. • Clearly communicate and display classroom expectations. • Be mindful of how you issue consequences (e.g., your tone of voice, body language).
Forgiven Without forgiveness, students come into class carrying the weight of their previous day's misbehavior.	• Say the words. While many of us forgive our students, we need to communicate that clearly (e.g., "I forgive you. We start over now.").

Now, you give it a try. Choose three keys to connection and brainstorm strategies to support students. **Hint:** How do you prefer others to connect with you?

Keys to Connection	Strategies

Want to know a quick connection hack? Laughter. Students love when teachers use humor. We all want to laugh and have fun. Sarcasm can be a well-intentioned attempt at connection. However, sarcasm is not always the most effective way to connect with students. The word *sarcasm* comes from the Greek *sarkasmós*, meaning "to tear flesh, bite the lip in rage, sneer." Yowza!

Also, sarcasm can be extremely difficult for English learners and students with learning disabilities to recognize and understand as humor. For younger students, sarcasm can also be very confusing and likely mimicked at inappropriate times.

Be mindful of any negative undertones, especially those directed at any one student. The benefit of potentially getting a quick laugh is never worth the cost of alienating a student. Students need to feel safe emotionally to engage in class.

Classroom Values

You can also use this Keys to Connection checklist by sharing it with your students! In groups, students can use sentence frames to share their thoughts and opinions. (You can differentiate this activity for younger students by modifying the list and incorporating visuals.)

Once students identify which feelings are most important to them personally, they can come together as a class to determine what they collectively value. Then they can create a poster to display in their classroom (see Figure 4.2). That way, whenever anyone behaves out of accordance with the collective values, they can be reminded and hold one another accountable.

Figure 4.2: Classroom Values

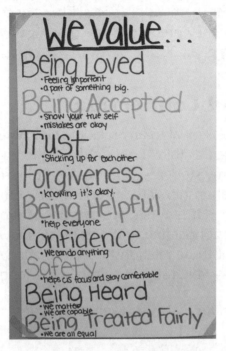

Students loved this activity because they really valued being able to cocreate and contribute to a sense of classroom identity. Decision-making activities during which all students have a say contribute to creating an equitable, student-centered classroom.

Connecting Across Cultures

To truly connect with students, we need to be aware of and respect their perspectives, cultures, languages, and differences. Building meaningful relationships with all students means understanding who they are at their core. Language and culture are essential to our identities. Stakeholders who are culturally and linguistically responsive create more meaningful, sustaining connections with students. As you might remember from earlier chapters, cultural and linguistic responsiveness (CLR) is the validation and affirmation of indigenous (home) culture and language, with the purpose of building and bringing students into success in the culture of academia and mainstream society (Hollie 2018). When we validate and affirm students around these essential aspects of their identities, they feel seen, heard, and valued. Why is this so important? We know from research that students are better able to learn and take risks when they feel emotionally safe and when they feel their cultures and languages are a valued part of their school community. We support our students, families, and communities best when we communicate messages of respect and acceptance. In contrast, anxiety and toxic stress are created by negative stereotypes, biases, unfair discipline practices, and other exclusionary or shaming practices. These become impediments to learning because they preoccupy the brain with worry and fear (Darling-Hammond et al. 2021).

Home-School Connections

Communication is essential to any relationship. When I was a high school teacher, I used to think I did not have the time to communicate personally with all my students, but I realized that making an investment in a relationship with a student early on pays dividends throughout the year. Oftentimes, we cite lack of time as the thing that keeps us from truly connecting and getting to know our students. What we find is that these relationships make our lives and our jobs easier—not harder—which saves us time in the long run!

Take a look at this note that was given to a student.

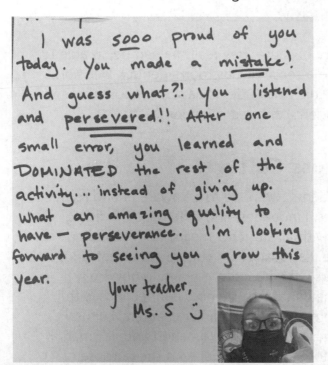

Notes build relationships.

This is also a fantastic example of how to encourage a growth mindset by giving specific and meaningful praise.

Personal Reflection

How long do you think it took this teacher to write this note? What kind of impact do you think it had on the student?

Positive Phone Calls Home

The simple act of calling home is one of the most effective relationship-building strategies, especially during remote learning. We have heard many heartwarming stories and received such positive feedback from teachers, students, and parents. Parents have shared that hearing something kind about their children "made their week." In turn, the student's good behavior is acknowledged and positively reinforced.

This practice also helps "flip the script" on students who have become accustomed to teachers reaching out to their parents or guardians for disciplinary reasons. During those points of contact with parents, our connection with the student is likely strained. We understand now more than ever, connecting with students in a virtual setting can be especially challenging. One way to connect with students *and* parents is to make positive phone calls home. You can "catch" the student doing something positive and call home. And since many students might not have a mom or dad at home, we like to use the word "adult."

"Tasha, thank you so much for sharing today. Who is the adult that I can call to share how much I appreciate your participation?"

Storytime

My eighth-grade teacher, Mrs. Montgomery, was my favorite teacher of all time. She believed in me, challenged me, and took the time to help me after school. She called me a "good writer." She was passionate about teaching. Her passion was contagious. After eighth grade graduation, I lost track of her. However, I thought about her often. I went on to become a bilingual teacher—just like her. I even went on to teach in her classroom in my former school. Later, when I moved to Los Angeles to teach at USC, I shared stories about Mrs. Montgomery with my students.

In the summer of 2019, I was about to walk out on stage in front of an auditorium of Chicago Public School teachers when I looked out into the audience and saw none other than Mrs. Montgomery.

Naturally, I freaked out and cried and told everyone the story. Mrs. Montgomery (now Dr. Montgomery) and I hugged and cried. Twenty-three years later, I finally got to tell my favorite teacher just how big of an impact she had on my life.

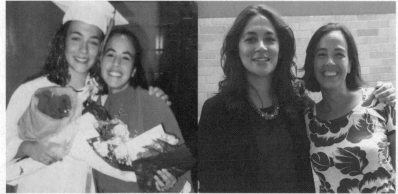

Trisha DiFazio with Dr. Montgomery in 1995

Trisha DiFazio with Dr. Montgomery in 2019

The moral of the story: Relationships matter (and also, Dr. Montgomery DID NOT age). Teaching is hard work, but every single day we are given the opportunity to be someone's Mrs. Montgomery.

Chapter Summary

One of the most important and rewarding things educators can do is build and maintain healthy relationships with their students. Students flourish socially and academically when they feel they are connected to their teachers and peers. Connection provides us all an elevated sense of well-being. Adults create meaningful connections with students when we affirm and promote the understanding of our students' identities, values, languages, and cultures.

Discussion Questions

1. What are your biggest takeaways from this chapter?

2. How can you apply the knowledge you have gained from this chapter?

3. Which aspects of relationship skills are you interested in learning more about?

Chapter 5: Responsible Decision-Making

What Is Responsible Decision-Making?

Pizza or tacos? Both—final answer. We make hundreds of choices a day, one after the other, about everything under the sun. Given how many decisions we make over the course of our lives, we say, let's get good at it.

But first, guess what plays a huge role in the choices we make? Our feelings. Talk about a full-circle moment! It is always helpful to take a moment to label our emotions and consider how they may be influencing our decisions. Using other SEL competencies to get in touch with our own feelings on matters (self-awareness), cool down our brains to make more rational decisions (self-management), or understand how our actions will impact others (social awareness) all help us make better decisions.

CASEL defines *responsible decision-making* as "the abilities to make caring and constructive choices about personal behavior and social interactions across diverse situations." This includes the capacity to consider ethical standards and safety concerns and to evaluate the benefits and consequences of various actions for personal, social, and collective well-being. One who demonstrates responsible decision-making can:

- demonstrate curiosity and open-mindedness
- learn how to make a reasoned judgment after analyzing information, data, and facts
- identify solutions for personal and social problems
- anticipate and evaluate the consequences of one's actions
- recognize how critical-thinking skills are useful both inside and outside of school
- reflect on one's role to promote personal, family, and community well-being
- evaluate personal, interpersonal, community, and institutional impacts

Why Is Responsible Decision-Making Important?

Our brains are not fully developed until around age 25. Those of us over 25 rely on the prefrontal cortex (the "rational" part of the brain) to make sound, responsible decisions. As previously mentioned, research shows children, teens, and young adults use the "emotional" or "reactionary" part of the brain to make decisions and often base their judgements on their emotions rather than considering long-term consequences (Rockwell 2019; Stanford Children's Health n.d.). We realize this may not come as a surprise to anyone who has spent time with a young person.

> "A moment of patience in a moment of anger saves you a hundred moments of regret."
>
> —Miguel Ruiz

Making sound decisions is difficult when we are angry, tired, hungry, dehydrated, or feeling challenged. Self-care habits and self-management skills will help us make better decisions. In addition, we can learn how to evaluate the benefits and consequences of our actions rather than simply acting on emotion. Participating in a decision-making process with intention helps build capacity to make choices that best serve ourselves and others. In doing so, we are reinforcing our ability to *respond* (pause, evaluate consequences, and make a constructive decision that considers all parties involved) rather than *react*.

 ## Personal Reflection

When you were young, what helped you make good decisions? What helps you make good decisions now? What's most difficult for you about making decisions?

Many young people do not realize just how many options they have in a given situation. The methods and strategies shared in this chapter will help students understand that the more options they explore, the better their final decisions are likely to be. And just like most SEL skills, it will take time and practice.

Responsible Decision-Making in the Classroom

Students can practice responsible decision-making in a low-stakes way through classroom activities that you design.

Would You Rather...?

One simple strategy to get your students started with decision-making is by playing, "Would You Rather...?" This is an easy, fun, low-stakes activity that gets your students' neurons firing around decision-making. You can incorporate kinesthetic learning by having students walk to the side of the room that represents their decision or simply raise their hands. Then, have the students share how and why they made their choices. It is also engaging when you let students change their decisions, switch sides, and provide their rationales.

As students become better acquainted with this strategy, you can make the questions more challenging and incorporate time for students to do any additional research.

Do you prefer dogs or cats? Why?

Would you rather have the ability to fly or be invisible?

Would you rather get $100 a week or $500 a month? Why?

Would you rather be the president of the United States or a Supreme Court justice? Why?

The frameworks below can be used to enhance the decision-making in playing "Would You Rather...?" and are practical tools for creating the "pause" to evaluate consequences and make constructive decisions in any area of the student's life.

Decision Tree

A decision tree is a flowchart-like graphic to provide visual representations of possible outcomes for our decisions. This strategy makes what can be an abstract process more concrete for students as they think through, write, and see the decision-making process unfold. Have the student bring a real-life example they are thinking about or that has been challenging them recently. For example, if the student has not been going to school (or showing up on video), you can use a decision tree to illustrate options and likely outcomes for attending or not attending class.

Using Figure 5.1 below as an example, the student would write *Class* in the biggest box at the top, and in the branches immediately below, they would write *not going to class* and *going to class*. Under each corresponding "branch," you and the student can fill in the likely consequences of going to class and not going to class. You are welcome to add as many branches to the tree as you'd like.

Figure 5.1: Decision Tree Example

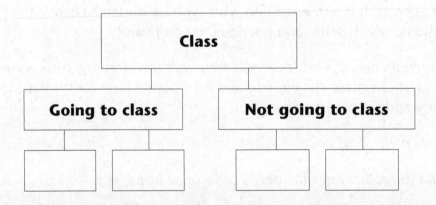

Connect Choices Now with Future Goals

Seeing the connection between the choices we make now and how they impact our future goals helps us make better decisions. To be effective, it is helpful to first have future goals. Ask students to make lists of their favorite classes, hobbies, and other preferred activities. Have students consider career opportunities of interest that align with their lists. Give students time to research the education, training, and other commitments involved with their career choices. Discuss how the choices they make today will impact their future goals (both positively and negatively) (Rockwell 2019).

Using Reflection in Decision-Making

We do not always make the right decisions. In fact, oftentimes we learn the biggest lessons when we make bad decisions. Make sure you give your students freedom to make mistakes, and create an open and safe space to reflect on those mistakes. Decision-making grows stronger when students can navigate challenging situations on their own.

 ## SEL in Action

Here are some specific questions you can ask students to support reflection on their decision-making.

- What's the last big mistake you made?
- What did you learn from it?
- How was that important to you?
- How did your decision impact the future?

Empathy in Decision-Making

Another useful practice is using empathy skills (from the social awareness competency) to take the opposing viewpoint in the decision-making process so the student has a greater understanding of the various perspectives and potential outcomes. Similarly, there is an opportunity for students to be more understanding and empathetic with themselves. We all have an inner dialogue or inner critic. When we are hard on ourselves, our inner critic often has us disengage with school and activities. We might lose connection with others, which is often, ironically, what we need most in those moments. One way to bring awareness to being more empathetic with ourselves is to ask, "What advice would you give a friend?" or "How would you talk to a friend or loved one about this?" These are great ways for students to tap into their "inner wisdom" on a topic and to notice the difference in the way they talk to themselves versus the way they would talk to someone else. Often, we would never talk to another person the way we talk to ourselves!

Incorporate Ethics and Morals into Decision-Making

There are several factors that impact our decision-making, some of which can be useful and some of which can get in the way. Bias, the natural human tendency to favor one thing over another, can get in the way of making good decisions. Supporting students in increasing their self-awareness to examine their own beliefs and biases will bolster their ability to make ethical and socially responsible decisions.

Introducing ethical dilemmas in the classroom can open up opportunities not only for debate and critical thinking but also for personal growth, empathy for other viewpoints, and self-reflection because students learn to navigate their own moral decision-making (Lee 2019). Use academic content to challenge your students to think critically about their own morals and ethics. For example, examining and discussing the roles of historical figures and characters from novels, as well as people involved with current events, can provide valuable teaching moments.

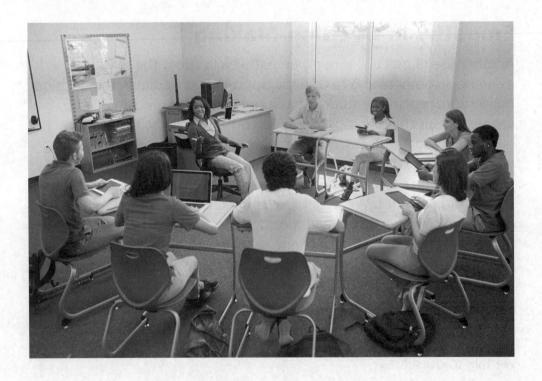

Spotlight

One of my students was caught texting in the hallway. When a teacher asked him to turn the phone over, he bolted. This resulted in a three-day suspension versus just picking up his phone at the end of the day. I went to see him and discuss what had happened. He was clearly not happy with the outcome, so we walked through what he could have done differently. That's when I realized he hadn't weighed the outcomes of his decisions. He experienced a literal "fight or flight" situation, and he ran. It was clear that no one had ever walked him through the decision-making process; he ran because he didn't know that he had other options.

I learned two SEL lessons that day. First, without a real conversation, assigning consequences is worthless. My student thought his punishment was unfair and didn't see how he could have made a different choice. Second, this is a story about next time. There is an inherent hopefulness in next time. Kids need to believe you will be there for them the next time. This time isn't going to end your relationship. And the reality is, many kids will face these same choices again, and they need help making better decisions.

—Kim Carlton
Educational Consultant
Dallas, Texas

Chapter Summary

Responsible decision-making is a lifelong skill that can create positive outcomes in our lives. Giving students opportunities to make decisions using real-life scenarios strengthens critical-thinking skills and promotes self- and social awareness. Using intentional support around decision-making-like frameworks and organizers helps make this abstract process more concrete. The goal is to guide students to build their capacity and incorporate skills from the other competencies to ultimately make responsible decisions.

Discussion Questions

1. What are your biggest takeaways from this chapter?

2. How can you apply the knowledge you have gained from this chapter?

3. What aspects of responsible decision-making are you interested in learning more about?

Chapter 6: Mindfulness

"Between stimulus and response there is a space. In that space lies our freedom and our power to choose our response. In our response lies our growth and our happiness."

—Anonymous

What Is Mindfulness?

Mindfulness is paying attention to the present moment without judgement. It is one of the most effective, easy, and inexpensive ways to decrease stress and anxiety, improve interpersonal relationships, and strengthen compassion. Anyone that has ever practiced mindfulness can tell you that it is not always as easy as it sounds. Oftentimes, it is our chattering minds that are responsible for taking us out of the present moment and creating "mental noise" that can cause stress. For example, when we worry, we are focusing our thoughts on the future, which we cannot control. When we dwell, we are focusing our attention on the past, which we cannot change. This ties into personal agency because the only moment we really have control over is the present.

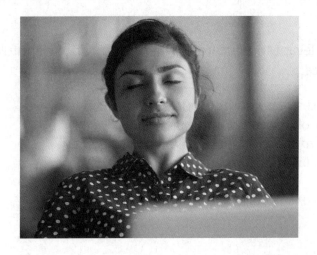

However, it turns out that we spend most of our time anywhere but in the present moment. In fact, a Harvard study found that people spend 46.9 percent of their waking hours thinking about something other than what they are doing (Eisler 2019). Whether we are driving, cleaning, or even in the middle of a conversation, our minds are often elsewhere, thinking about other things. When you are mindful, you are actively involved in the activity with all your senses, in the present moment, gently bringing yourself back to the conversation or task at hand instead of allowing your mind to wander (Eisler 2019).

While meditation and mindfulness are sometimes used interchangeably, they are not the same thing. Meditation typically refers to a formal seated practice for a specific amount of time, whereas mindfulness can be practiced anytime, anywhere, and applied to any situation throughout the day.

You can't stop the waves, but you can learn to surf."

—Jon Kabat-Zinn (1994)

Why Is Mindfulness Important?

Research indicates that mindfulness provides us with skills to build attention, improve focus, regulate emotions, and manage stress, allowing us to feel nourished and energized to support and connect with students in the classroom, at home, and beyond (Mindful Schools n.d.).

Particularly relevant to educators, when we practice mindfulness, we can experience:

- reduced stress and burnout
- greater efficacy in doing our jobs
- more emotionally supportive classrooms
- better classroom organization

Integrating SEL and Mindfulness

Here's how mindfulness is integrated into each of the competencies:

- **Self-awareness:** Students' self-awareness is enhanced by mindfulness practices that promote self-compassion and self-exploration.

- **Self-management:** Mindfulness increases students' emotion-regulation skills, which enhances their ability to *respond* rather than *react*.

- **Social Awareness:** Mindfulness increases students' empathy by helping them to regulate their emotions rather than get emotionally overwhelmed when faced with difficult situations.

- **Relationship Skills:** Mindfulness increases emotional awareness. People feel more comfortable interacting with individuals who are emotionally regulated.

- **Decision-making:** Mindfulness increases cognitive flexibility and creativity, which gives students a wider range of options when faced with difficult decisions. When we pause we give ourselves time and space to respond in a more intentional way.

Personal Reflection

Have you ever practiced mindfulness? If so, what was it like for you?

Breathing Strategies

We have a "life hack" that helps us regulate our physical, emotional, and mental state. Can you guess what it is? **Hint:** It is something we all have but is easily taken for granted. It is our ability to breathe. Humans typically take about 20,000 breaths each day. In moments when you feel stressed, anxious, or upset, focusing on breathing or changing the way you breathe can help de-escalate an intense moment and lower overall stress levels. Breathing techniques can greatly help calm the body and brain in just a few minutes. Teaching students these breathing practices supports emotional awareness from an early age, which ultimately strengthens social and emotional skills and helps children grow to be strong, healthy, compassionate people.

Here are a few breathing techniques for adults and students:

Smell the Roses, Blow Out the Birthday Candles

This is a great introduction for showing younger students how to manage and control their breathing. Have students inhale as if they are "smelling roses" and then exhale as if they are "blowing out the candles" on a birthday cake.

Dragon Breathing

Students love one of the most popular mythological creatures—dragons. Getting to "breathe like a dragon" is a great technique for releasing tension associated with anger. How to do it: Breathe in deeply though your nose. Hold. On the exhale, open your eyes and your mouth wide and stick out your tongue. Students can even hold up their "talons" (hands).

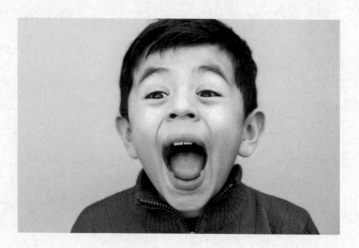

Switch Breath (Alternate Nostril Breathing)

Alternate nostril breathing can help reduce anxiety as well as relax your body and mind. It is also a quick and efficient practice that can be done before high-stress situations. How to do it: Close one nostril, and inhale for five seconds. Close the other nostril, and exhale for five seconds. Repeat.

Breathe and Count

This is a very simple breathing technique your students can use to calm their nervous systems and focus their brains in the heat of the moment or when they're feeling anxious. How to do it: Breathe in for four seconds, having the student count each second, and then exhale for four seconds. Work up to eight seconds, and change the inhale and exhale numbers (they do not have to match).

We have heard people say these exercises make them feel "more relaxed," "less tense," "energized," and even "playful." Give one of these techniques a try, and see what you notice!

Chapter Summary

We sometimes forget that one of our most effective coping mechanisms is an internal one. There are a multitude of benefits to practicing mindfulness. Incorporating mindfulness practices enhances and strengthens SEL skills. At the end of the day, we all benefit from being a little more present and a little less stressed. When in doubt, just breathe. You've got this.

Discussion Questions

1. What are your biggest takeaways from this chapter?

2. How can you apply the knowledge you have gained from this chapter?

3. What aspects of mindfulness are you interested in learning more about?

Chapter 7: SEL Activities

Competency Connections

The activities presented on the following pages are meant to provide options for intentionally addressing certain competencies. You'll notice that there is a lot of overlap in the competencies—that's because they are all interconnected!

Use these activities with your class when you want to intentionally put SEL skills into practice. They can be revisited throughout the year and adapted to situational needs. Creating a regular routine of SEL activities will reinforce these skills and underscore the importance of social and emotional learning.

Note: Each activity is designed to empower and connect with students. There are multiple opportunities within each activity to validate and celebrate students' languages, cultures, and identities.

Suggested sentence frames are provided. Feel free to differentiate these sentence frames for your students' language proficiency levels.

Activity	Integrated Competencies				
	Self-Awareness	Self-Management	Social Awareness	Relationship Skills	Responsible Decision-Making
Heart Art					
Name That Emotion					
"What Helps Me" Wheel					
Calming Countdown					
Perspective Detective					
What's Their Story?					
Who's My Crew?					
Keys to Connection					
Introduce Your Selfie/ Identity Slides					
SODAS					
T-Chart					

Heart Art

Grade Levels: K–5

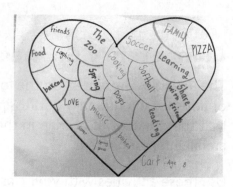

Target Competency
• Self-Awareness
Integrated Competencies
• Social Awareness
• Relationship Skills

Purpose

Help students identify what they love and value. Create connections between classmates and teachers by sharing their finished projects. This is a quick and easy way for students to feel seen and heard.

Materials

- *Heart Art* (page 113)
- digital heart outline or drawing application (*optional, for online instruction*)
- crayons, markers, or other drawing utensils
- sentence frames written on chart paper or on the board

Procedure

1. Provide students with copies of *Heart Art* or with instructions to draw their own hearts.

2. Tell students that they are going to do a self-awareness activity to help them learn more about themselves.

3. Explain that this activity will also help you get to know them better.

4. Discuss what it means when we love or value something.

5. Show an example of your own completed Heart Art project. Share what you love and value, and model using the sentence frames as you share.

6. Invite students to draw or write what they love and value in their heart outlines.

7. After students have completed their Heart Art projects, have students work with partners to share their hearts.

8. Remind students how to treat one another with kindness and respect while sharing their projects.

9. While students are sharing with each other, make sure to validate their willingness to share and participate.

10. When students are finished, ask reflection questions.

Specific Grade Level SEL Sentence Frames

Grades K–2

Provide a word wall to help students write new vocabulary. Students can also draw pictures of what they love.

> "I love _____."

> "What makes me happy is _____."

> "It's fun to _____."

Grades 3–5

Encourage students to use grade-level vocabulary. Have students brainstorm words, or provide a word bank to help them get started.

> "I value _____ because _____."

> "I love _____ because _____."

> "_____ is important to me because _____."

Student Reflection Questions

What did you like about this activity? What did you learn about a classmate?

Opportunities for Differentiation

- Support English learners by allowing them to describe or label the hearts in their home languages.

- Differentiate this activity by using different shapes. For example, mouse ears or a smiley face.

- Challenge students by using more rigorous vocabulary.

- Expand the lesson by having students find classmates with similarities and differences in their hearts.

- Integrate the arts by having students act out the things that they love.

 # Between Us

- This has the potential to be a highly vulnerable activity; allow students the freedom to pass on sharing verbally.

- Celebrate students' ability to share, and give specific and meaningful feedback about what they've created. For example: "Thanks for sharing that you love your mom's cooking. What's your favorite dish?" or "Nathan loves *Fortnite*. Does anyone else have that in common with him?"

- This activity could be fun to revisit later in the school year so students can see how they've grown and what's changed.

- Validate aspects of students' identities such as languages, cultures, etc.

Name: _____   Date:_____

Heart Art

Directions: Draw or write what you love and value in the heart outline.

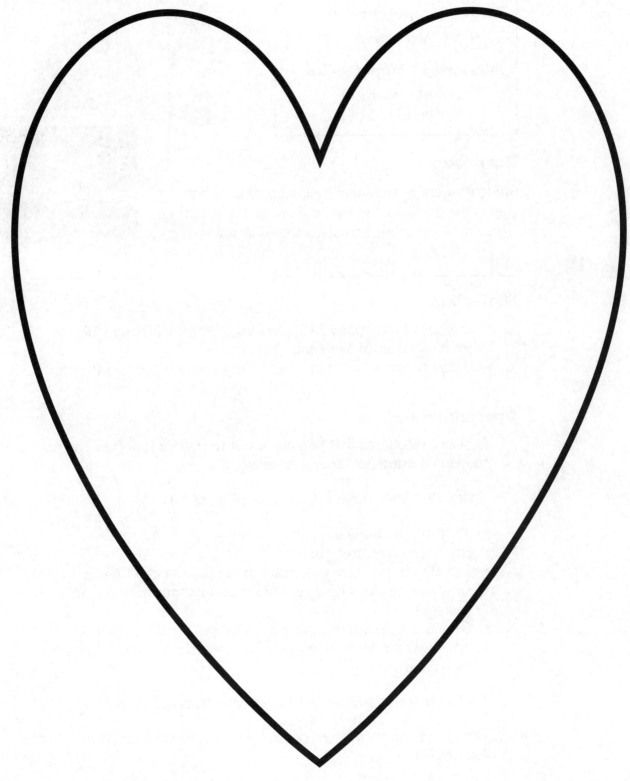

Name That Emotion

Grade Levels: K–12

Emotions Faces

Target Competency
- Self-Awareness

Integrated Competencies
- Self-Management
- Relationship Skills

Emotions Word Wheel

Emotions Word List

angry	depressed	isolated	happy
frustrated	anxious	abandoned	content
disgusted	stressed	embarrassed	comfortable
sad	confused	ashamed	excited
disappointed	hurt	lonely	confident

Purpose

Students identify and label their emotions, giving them time and space to better manage the resulting behavior—one of the first steps to self-awareness.

Materials

- *Emotions Faces* (page 118), *Emotions Word List* (page 119), or *Emotions Word Wheel* (page 120)
- sentence frames written on chart paper or on the board

Procedure

1. Explain to students that you are about to share a tool they can use to help describe how they are feeling.

2. Share, "We know several things about emotions:

   - All emotions are OK.
   - Emotions come and go.
   - Sometimes, we have more than one emotion at a time.
   - Emotions give us important information about how we are feeling.
   - Emotions help us communicate what we need.
   - When we can identify and label our emotions, we can better manage them."

3. Explain that this skill will get better with practice.

4. Display *Emotions Faces, Emotions Word List,* or *Emotions Word Wheel* for students.

Specific Grade Level SEL Sentence Frames

Grades K–2

Have students look at each face on *Emotions Faces* and describe what they think that person is feeling. How do they know? Have students use sentence frames to describe how they are feeling in the moment.

> "I think they feel _____ because _____."

Grades 3–5

Have students refer to the *Emotions Word List* and use sentence frames to identify their feelings in various scenarios.

Example: *Sometimes, I feel <u>nervous</u> when <u>I am called on in class</u>.*

Have students identify what happens to them physically when they feel different emotions.

Example: *I know I am feeling <u>worried</u> when my <u>stomach hurts</u>.*

> "Sometimes, I feel _____ when _____."

> "I know I am feeling _____ when my _____."

Grades 6–12

Have students refer to the *Emotions Word Wheel* and use sentence frames to identify and express their feelings in various scenarios. It is OK to have them start with very basic and simple adjectives to describe their feelings and then build in more complex vocabulary over time.

Example: *Sometimes, I feel <u>self-conscious</u> when <u>my teacher calls on me</u>.*

Have students identify what happens to them physically when they feel different emotions.

Example: *I know I am feeling <u>excited</u> when my <u>heart beats quickly</u>.*

> "Sometimes, I feel _____ when _____."

> "I know I am feeling _____ when my _____."

Student Reflection Questions

What did you learn about emotions? When is it helpful to name your emotions? What did you like about learning about emotions?

Opportunities for Differentiation

- Support English learners by providing them with written and visual supports.

- Challenge students by using more advanced emotion vocabulary.

- Gamify the lesson by playing charades with the emotions.

- Integrate the arts by having students draw their emotions.

- Adapt to an online format by using emojis.

- Have students make a set of cards for different emotions by cutting apart *Emotions Faces* (page 118) or *Emotions Word List* (page 119). Students can use them discreetly at their own desks to communicate what kind of day they are having without using words.

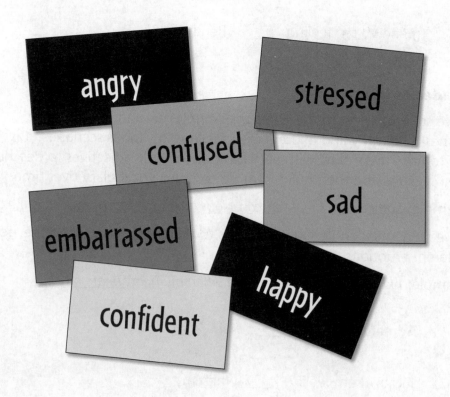

Between Us

- We do not want our students to feel shame around any of their feelings. Be open to all feelings shared by students, and be mindful of your own reactions when they are sharing. For example, if a student shares that they are angry, you may not have to fix anything in the moment; first, you can be there to listen.

- All feelings are valid for all students, regardless of gender.

- Practice, practice, practice. Mastery is achieved through repetition.

Name: _____ Date: _____

Emotions Faces

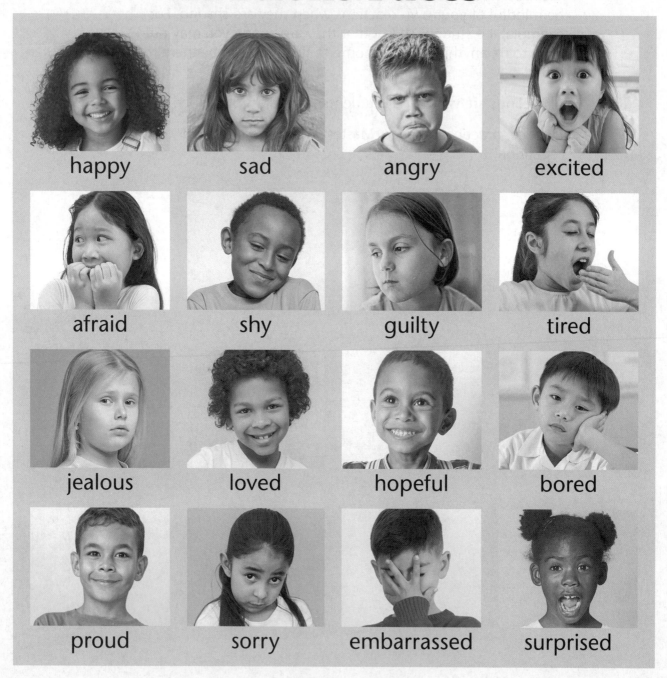

happy

sad

angry

excited

afraid

shy

guilty

tired

jealous

loved

hopeful

bored

proud

sorry

embarrassed

surprised

Emotions Word List

happy	isolated	depressed	angry
content	abandoned	anxious	frustrated
comfortable	embarrassed	stressed	disgusted
excited	ashamed	confused	sad
confident	lonely	hurt	disappointed

Emotions Word Wheel

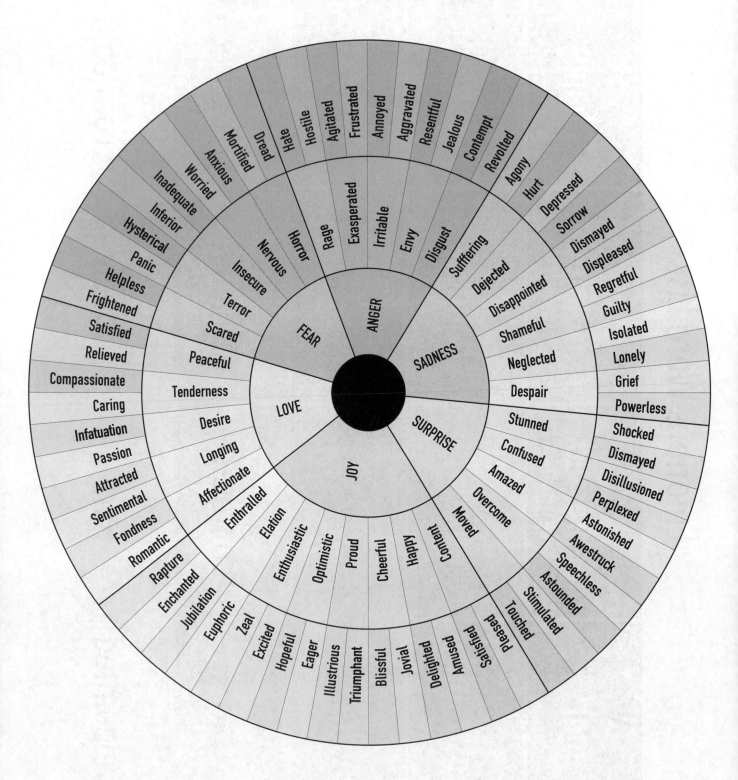

"What Helps Me" Wheel

Grade Levels: K–12

> **Target Competency**
> - Self-Management
>
> **Integrated Competencies**
> - Self-Awareness
> - Relationship Skills
> - Responsible Decision-Making

What Helps Me Wheel

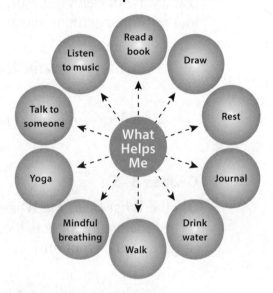

Purpose

Students identify the activities that help them feel better during times of stress. The wheel serves as a visual representation of their personal self-management tools.

Materials

- *What Helps Me Wheel* (pages 124, 125, 126; select the wheel that is appropriate for your students)
- sentence frames written on chart paper or on the board

Procedure

1. Explain that being self-aware includes understanding how to manage ourselves during times of stress. Share a completed wheel, and model how to use it.

2. Either as a whole-group or with partners, have students brainstorm the different types of activities that help them during challenging times.

3. Ask students to work independently to complete their own wheels.

4. Ask students how the wheels can help them throughout their day.

5. Encourage students to keep the wheels somewhere easily accessible.

6. Have students answer the reflection questions.

Specific Grade Level SEL Sentence Frames

Grades K–2

Use the *What Helps Me Wheel* on page 124 to help students identify four self-management activities.

> "(*Activity*) helps me feel better."

> "When I am upset, I like to _____."

Grades 3–5

Use the *What Helps Me Wheel* on page 125 to help students identify six self-management activities. Provide different options to help them target specific emotions.

> "When I am (*stressed, nervous, angry*), I can _____."

> "When I am (*upset, sad, lonely*), one way I can feel better is to _____."

Grades 6–12

Use the *What Helps Me Wheel* on page 126 to help students identify 10 self-management activities.

> "One activity that helps me when I am feeling _____ is _____."

> "One of my self-management tools is to _____."

Student Reflection Questions

When will the wheel come in handy for you? What did you learn about yourself?

Opportunities for Differentiation

- Support English learners by providing them with additional visual and textual supports.

- Expand the lesson by having students find classmates with similar activities in their wheels.

- Gamify this activity by having students play charades and act out the activities from their wheels.

- Connect to home by having students share their completed wheels with their parents/guardians.

- Adapt to online format by creating wheels digitally or using a storyboard app to animate their self-management strategies.

 # Between Us

- Make your own personal *What Helps Me Wheel*.

- Be sure to validate student responses.

- Support students to use these practices consistently.

Name: _____   Date:_____

What Helps Me Wheel

Directions: Draw or write about what helps you.

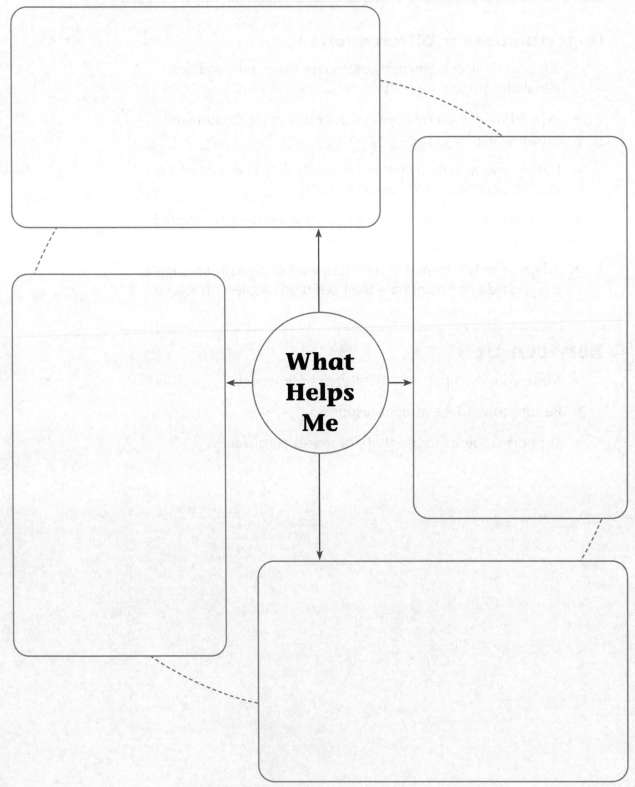

Name: _____ Date: _____

What Helps Me Wheel

Directions: Draw or write about what helps you.

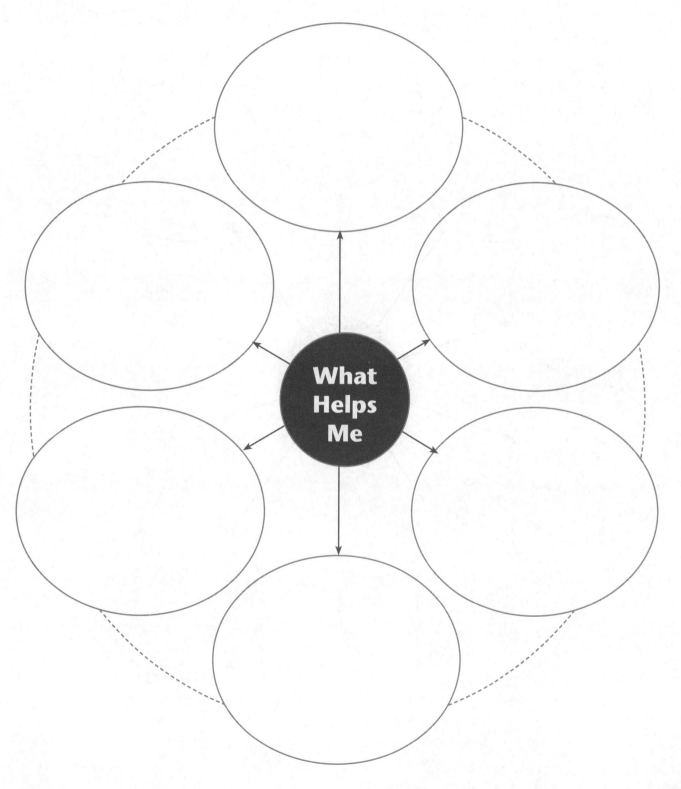

Name: _____ Date: _____

What Helps Me Wheel

Directions: Draw or write about what helps you.

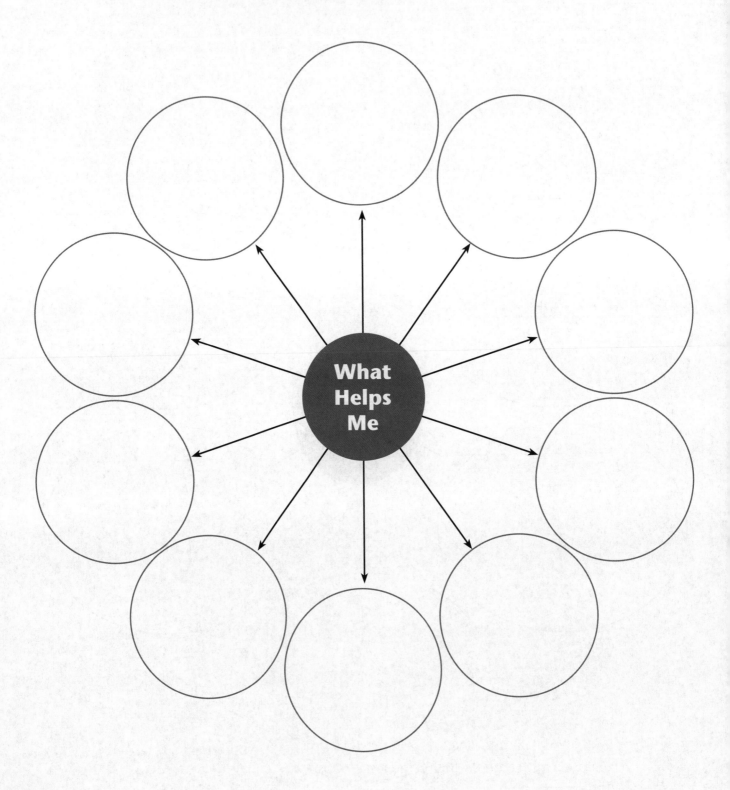

Calming Countdown

Grade Levels: K–12

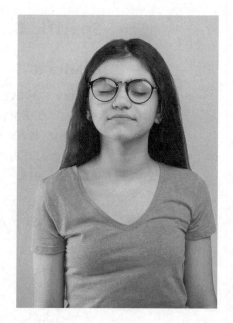

Target Competency
- Self-Management

Integrated Competencies
- Self-Awareness
- Responsible Decision-Making

Purpose

Students "cool down" their minds during moments of stress or anxiety. The practice of focusing your attention teaches emotional awareness and self-management.

Materials

- *Calming Countdown* (page 130)
- sentence frames written on chart paper or on the board

Preparation

- Familiarize yourself with this strategy by practicing a few times before introducing it to your students.

Procedure

1. Display the *Calming Countdown* poster.

2. Tell students that when we are stressed or upset, we can calm ourselves using tools we already have—our five senses.

3. Explain that focusing on our five senses is a simple and easy way to feel calm during moments of intense emotion.

4. Review the five senses: sight, sound, smell, touch, taste.

5. Model how to do the Calming Countdown. Think aloud through each question, letting students hear your answers. "What are five things I see?" and "I see a _____."

6. Ask students to practice the Calming Countdown by saying the answers silently to themselves.

7. When finished, ask students the reflection questions.

Specific Grade Level SEL Sentence Frames

Grades K–5

Review the five senses. As a group, brainstorm possible answers for each step. Post additional vocabulary words on the board for reference. The goal is for students to gradually be able to do this independently. A good visual and kinesthetic tool is to count off each of the five steps on your fingers.

> "My five senses are _____, _____, _____, _____, _____."

> "I see _____, _____, _____, _____, _____."

> "I hear _____, _____, _____, _____."

> "The Calming Countdown helped me to _____."

> "In the future, this strategy can help me to _____."

Grades 6–12

Discuss when students might feel stressed out or upset. Share that we can calm ourselves just by using our five senses. Discuss how using mindfulness/breathing apps could benefit students. Also, ask students if they would make any modifications to the countdown. It is an anxiety hack!

> "The Calming Countdown helped me to _____."

> "In the future, this strategy can help me to _____."

Student Reflection Questions

What did you like about this activity? When can you use this tool?

Opportunities for Differentiation

- Validate English learners by allowing them to give answers in their home languages.

- Integrate the arts by having younger students draw outlines of their hands and write the name of each sense on each of the fingers.

- Integrate technology by having older students make photo collages of items that relate to each sense. They can imagine these items as part of their Calming Countdown.

 # Between Us

- Model and practice as many times as needed.

- Remind students during the day that they can do the Calming Countdown on their own.

- Validate and praise students when they use self-management strategies.

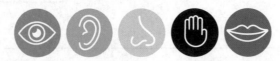

Calming Countdown

Identify in the moment

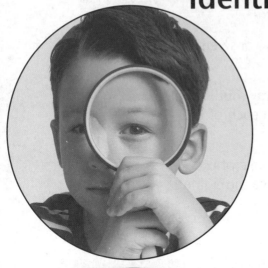

- five things you see

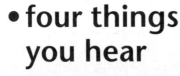

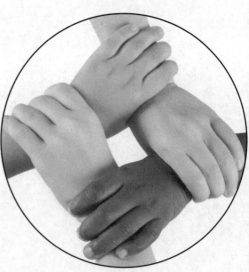

- four things you hear

- three things you smell

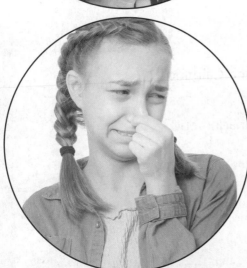

- two things you touch

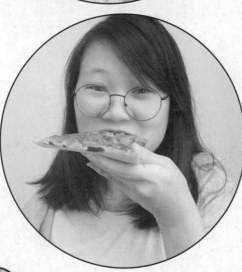

- one thing you taste

126898—Social-Emotional Learning Starts with Us

Perspective Detective

Grade Levels: K–12

Target Competency
- Social Awareness

Integrated Competencies
- Self-Awareness
- Self-Management
- Relationship Skills
- Responsible Decision-Making

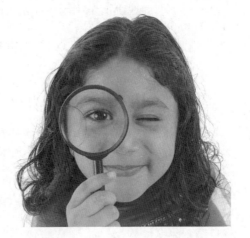

Purpose

Students adopt a different perspective and become more conscious of other people's feelings and experiences.

Materials

- *Perspective Detective Graphic Organizer Sample* (page 135) and *Perspective Detective Graphic Organizer* (page 136)
- supplemental visuals of the person or scenario selected
- sentence frames written on chart paper or on the board

Preparation

- Think of a fictional or historical person and a scenario they encountered.
- Gather and display any supplemental visuals of the person and the scenario (e.g., Ruby Bridges' first day of school).

Procedure

1. Define *empathy* and *perspective taking* (see Social Awareness chapter for definitions).

2. Explain that the goal of this activity is to relate to another person's perspective by thinking about their unique circumstances, experiences, beliefs, and culture.

3. Present the individual (living person, historical figure, character from book) and a scenario that person encountered. Use visuals as necessary to help students imagine the person.

4. Ask students questions that help them to examine that individual's thoughts, feelings, and behaviors.

5. Encourage students to use evidence as well as their imaginations to see things from that person's perspective.

6. Model how to complete the organizer, using the sample as needed.

7. Provide word banks for students (such as *Emotions Faces*, *Emotions Word List*, or *Emotions Word Wheel* on pages 118–120).

8. Use the completed *Perspective Detective Graphic Organizer* to respond to the reflection questions.

Specific Grade Level SEL Sentence Frames

Grades K–2

Share and model sentence frames so students feel comfortable sharing their perspectives. Make sure to include many visuals to help students relate to the experience.

"I think she feels _____."

"I think he feels _____."

"I think they feel _____ because _____."

Grades 3–5

Have students paint more vivid pictures of the circumstances surrounding the character's scenario by including a variety of visuals that may represent different emotions. Encourage students to use academic language and higher-level vocabulary. In future lessons, have students identify a person they would like to relate to from history, literature, or a current event.

"I think they feel _____ because _____."

"I would feel _____ because _____."

Grades 6–12

Have students choose more complex characters from more abstract sources, such as poetry, songs, or biographies. Encourage students to use academic language and higher-level vocabulary as they find textual evidence to support their ideas.

> "I think they feel _____ because _____."

> "The line that states '(*insert line from text*)' indicates that the character feels _____ because _____."

Student Reflection Questions

What did you learn about this person that you didn't know before? What is one way this has changed your own perspective?

Opportunities for Differentiation

- Empower students by allowing them to vote on who to choose for the activity.

- Support English learners by having students base this activity on a notable person who learned English as another language.

- Be culturally responsive by encouraging students to choose people with different linguistic or cultural backgrounds.

- Expand the activity by writing a letter from the perspective of the person being studied. Get creative by having students create fictional Twitter®, Facebook®, or Instagram® posts based on the character's perspective.

- Integrate the arts by having students draw comic strips and use thought bubbles to demonstrate the thoughts and feelings of the person. Or encourage role-playing, acting out sketches, or performing puppet shows.

Between Us

- Perspective-taking skills are especially important during cross-cultural interactions, as people likely have very different perceptions of the world. Be sure to encourage perspective taking when students are learning about other cultures or ways of life.

- Be sure to validate home languages and home cultures of both the students and the figures they have chosen.

- Be mindful that students may take on perspectives that could be uncomfortable for other students. Use your best judgement when selecting figures to do the Perspective Detective exercise.

Perspective Detective
Graphic Organizer Sample

Person/Name ⟶	Ruby Bridges
Situation ⟶	She was the first African American student to attend an all-white elementary school in the South.
When? ⟶	1960
Where? ⟶	Louisiana
What is happening? (Describe the situation.) ⟶	Ruby is standing outside the school, about to walk in for the first time. She and her mom are being escorted by four federal marshals.
How might the person be feeling? ⟶	scared, nervous, excited
Why do you think that? (Use evidence and your imagination.) ⟶	I think she might feel scared because four police officers had to escort her into the school. I think she was nervous because there was a crowd of people surrounding her. I think she might feel excited because it is her first day of her new school.
How would you feel? ⟶	scared, nervous, excited

Perspective Detective Graphic Organizer

Directions: Complete the chart with information and your ideas about the situation.

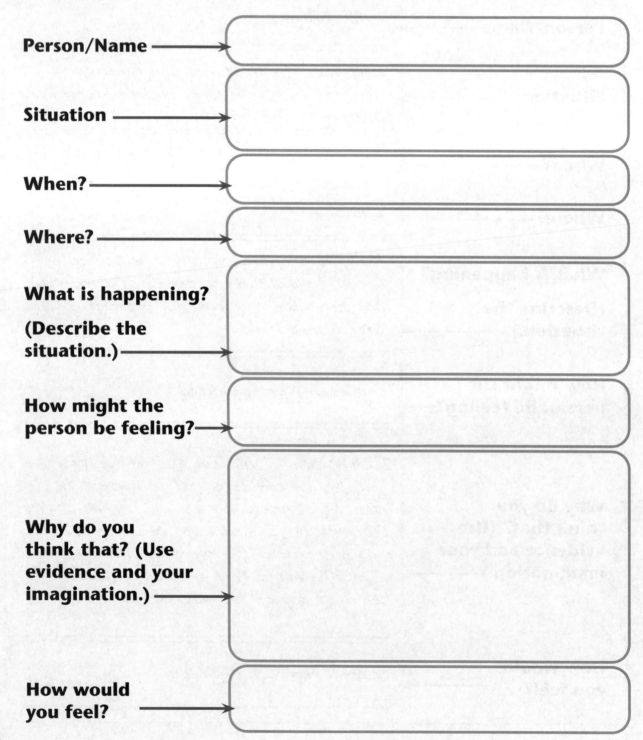

Person/Name ⟶

Situation ⟶

When? ⟶

Where? ⟶

What is happening?
(Describe the situation.) ⟶

How might the person be feeling? ⟶

Why do you think that? (Use evidence and your imagination.) ⟶

How would you feel? ⟶

What's Their Story?

Grade Levels: 3–12

Target Competency
- Social Awareness

Integrated Competency
- Relationship Skills

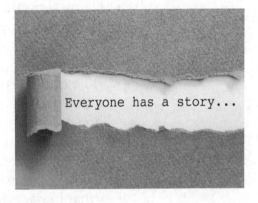

Everyone has a story...

Purpose

Students identify and evaluate how important events shape one's life. Students use research and empathy skills to build social awareness.

Materials

- paper, poster board, or instructions for digital platform
- drawing and coloring supplies
- sentence frames written on chart paper or on the board

Procedure

1. Share with students that this activity will help them learn more about others and the events that shaped their lives.

2. Have each student choose an individual about whose life they would like to learn more. This could be someone they know personally, a historical figure, or someone in the news. Explain that they will be creating a time line of important events and key milestones in that person's life.

3. Model with a completed time line example (see page 140), and think aloud to demonstrate creating a time line.

4. Use prompts to help students:

- Why did you choose this person?
- What is something you learned about them that surprised you?
- Name something you have in common with them.
- Name one way you are different from them.
- What would this person's hashtag be?
- Choose an important event.
- How do you think that event impacted their life?
- If this person were going to give you one piece of advice, what do you think it would be?
- If you were this person, would you do anything differently? Why?
- If you could ask them one question, what would it be?
- What impact do you think they had on those around them?

5. Have students work with small groups to present their completed time lines. In a digital environment, students can record their presentations and take turns watching them.

Specific Grade Level SEL Sentence Frames

Grades 3–5

Model expectations for how the small groups will work by demonstrating with students in front of the class.

> "I chose this person because _____."

> "Something that stands out to me about _____ is _____."

> "Something I found really interesting about _____ was _____."

Grades 6–12

Encourage the use of higher-order questions for students when appropriate.

> "An important event in _____'s life was when _____."

> "A difficult time in _____'s life was when _____."

> "If I were this person, I would _____."

> "Based on my research _____."

Student Reflection Questions

What did you like about this activity? What would you change about this activity? What did you learn about yourself?

Opportunities for Differentiation

- Support English learners by reinforcing vocabulary with visuals.

- Expand the lesson by having students choose from a menu of options: write a poem or song about the person; make a drawing; design an imaginary Twitter account.

- Integrate math by having students design math problems using numbers from the time line (e.g., use years and dates to show sequences).

- Integrate the arts by having students do first-person monologues.

- Adapt to online format by creating time lines digitally and using photos or online images.

- Expand the activity by creating and displaying a time line of historical events, and have students put their character's time lines alongside world events. This can provide context and may help students see a different perspective.

Between Us

- Feel free to augment this lesson with your own personal teacher flair.

- Validate student participation in the small groups.

- This activity may be completed over several days.

What's Their Story? Time Line Example

Date	Event
July 12, 1997	**The Birth of Malala** Malala Yousafzai is born on July 12, 1997 in Mingora, Pakistan.
September 1, 2008	**First Speech** Malala Yousafzai at age 11, gives a speech in front of the national press—"How Dare the Taliban Take Away My Basic Right to an Education?"
January 6, 2009	**A Fake Name** Malala starts blogging for BBC Urdu in January 2009 using the pseudonym (a fake name), Gul Makai.
October 9, 2012	**Assassination Attempt** Malala is shot while traveling home from school by a Taliban gunman.
October 9, 2013	**Book Published** Malala's memoir *I Am Malala* is released.
October 10, 2014	**Nobel Peace Prize** Malala wins Nobel Peace Prize
October 2, 2015	**Movie** Malala's documentary titled *He Named Me Malala* is released in theaters.

Who's My Crew?

Grade Levels: K–12

Target Competency
- Social Awareness

Integrated Competencies
- Self-Management
- Relationship Skills
- Responsible Decision-Making

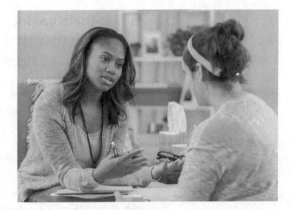

Purpose

Students identify individuals, groups, and organizations where they can get support.

Materials

- *Who's My Crew?* (page 145)
- sentence frames written on chart paper or on the board

Preparation

- Be prepared to share examples of your own "crew."
- Gather contact information of staff members, groups, or organizations within the school and community to provide as examples for students.

Procedure

1. Share that the goal of this activity is to help students identify and locate people, groups, or organizations they can go to when they need help.

2. Distribute *Who's My Crew?* to students. Explain that *crew* is referring to the adults (e.g., counselor, coach, nurse, neighbor, caseworker/case manager, family members) who can support and help them.

3. Discuss the value of identifying who is in their crew.

4. Provide students time to reflect on their own.

5. Have students complete the *Who's My Crew* page, identifying individuals or organizations in their lives that they can go to for support.

Specific Grade Level SEL Sentence Frames

Grades K–2

Explain that there are lots of places and people students can go to when they need help. Model by thinking aloud and providing an example. Encourage students to use sentence frames.

> "_____ is someone I can go to if I'm feeling sad."

> "_____ is someone I can go to if I need help."

> "_____ is someone I can go to if I have questions."

Grades 3–5

Encourage students to start to identify resources not only in their immediate environment but those within the community as well. If students have cell phones, they can program important numbers into their phones. Students can also write who is in their crew on sheets of paper as a reference.

> "_____ is someone I can go to if I have a question or concern."

> "_____ is someone I can count on."

> "_____ is someone I like talking to when I am worried."

> "_____ is someone who can help me solve a problem."

Grades 6–12

Encourage students to identify resources beyond their immediate environment, within the greater community. Support students to stretch a bit and think outside the box as to who might be in their crew. If students have cell phones, they can program important numbers into their phones or store them on cards in their wallets or purses. If students do not have the school counselor or other school support services listed, consider inviting that person to class to remind students of the support offered in school.

For eleventh and twelfth graders, expand the discussion of "Who's My Crew?" into networking opportunities so students can think about who to connect with for college, employment opportunities, financial aid, or summer internships.

> "For help with (*college, financial aid, wellness*), I can go to _____."

> "I can find information about _____ by asking _____ or by looking up _____ online."

> "A good resource to find help with _____ is _____."

> "_____ is someone who would be helpful to have on my team in the future."

Student Reflection Questions

What's one thing you like about seeing who's in your crew? What might you do with this knowledge moving forward?

Opportunities for Differentiation

- Expand the activity by having the students contact the individuals they have identified to let them know they are in their crew.

- Support English learners by helping them identify English translation services that may be available at the school or within a community organization for themselves or their families.

- Integrate the arts by having students design business cards with contact info of their crew.

- Extend the activity by having students identify people that would be helpful to add to their crew in the future. This might include adults within the school or in their community (e.g., guidance counselor, coach, religious leader).

- Enhance this activity by spotlighting a school resource employee each month and having them be a guest speaker in your class. Then, display a poster of that person with their contact information.

Between Us

- No student's crew should be empty. Support them to identify at least two adults.

- This is not meant to be a "best friend competition," which is why the focus should be on adult support rather than peers.

- Keep this information between you and the student. It does not need to be shared publicly in class.

Name: _____ Date: _____

Who's My Crew?

Directions: Complete the chart with people and places you can go to for support.

My Crew	Name	Can Help With	Contact Information
Individual			
Individual			
Group/Team			
Group/Team			
Organization			
Organization			

Keys to Connection

Grade Levels: 3–12

Target Competency
- Relationship Skills

Integrated Competencies
- Self-Awareness
- Self-Management
- Social Awareness

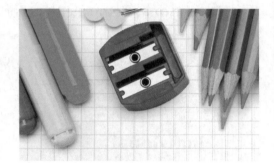

Purpose

Students identify how to establish connections and develop positive relationships.

Materials

- *Keys to Connection Checklist* (page 149)
- chart paper, one sheet for each small group
- markers for each group
- sentence frames written on chart paper or on the board

Preparation

- Display sentence frames.

Procedure

1. Explain that having positive relationships helps us all feel connected to one another.

2. Share the *Keys to Connection Checklist*, and review terms.

3. Define any unfamiliar vocabulary, and provide examples.

4. Have students collaborate in small groups to choose five keys that are most important to them, and record the words on chart paper.

5. Groups select a presenter to share their answers.

6. Have students complete the reflection questions independently.

Specific Grade Level SEL Sentence Frames

Grades 3–5

Use a modified list of connection vocabulary words. Make sure students understand the meaning of all the words before you begin the lesson.

> "It is important to me that I feel _____ in a relationship because _____."

> "I feel _____ in a relationship when _____."

> "I do not feel _____ when _____."

Grades 6–12

Emphasize the importance of students being able to justify their thinking. Feel free to extend this lesson over multiple class periods.

> "I want my teacher to know _____."

> "In my opinion, I think _____ is important because _____."

> "I value _____ because _____."

> "While I understand _____'s point, I think _____."

Student Reflection Questions

What did you learn about yourself that you did not know before? What did you learn about your classmates? What did you like about this activity?

Opportunities for Differentiation

- Support English learners by providing them with visual and written supports.

- Expand the lesson by compiling individual answers to create a Classroom Values poster. Turn this into a Classroom Contract for group or classroom accountability.

- Incorporate math by creating a bar graph of student choices.

- Gamify this activity by having students create a gesture for each word and then playing charades.

Between Us

- There are no right or wrong answers. The power is in the students sharing their voices and being validated by adults and their peers.

- Give students specific and meaningful praise when working in groups and sharing their ideas.

- Step back and let your students take the wheel on this one.

- This list can be used many ways, so feel free to get creative with it.

Keys to Connection Checklist

- ☐ accepted
- ☐ acknowledged
- ☐ admired
- ☐ appreciated
- ☐ approved of
- ☐ believed in
- ☐ capable
- ☐ challenged
- ☐ competent
- ☐ confident
- ☐ forgiven
- ☐ heard
- ☐ helpful
- ☐ important
- ☐ included
- ☐ in control
- ☐ listened to
- ☐ loved

- ☐ needed
- ☐ noticed
- ☐ respected
- ☐ safe
- ☐ supported
- ☐ treated fairly
- ☐ trusted
- ☐ understood
- ☐ useful
- ☐ validated
- ☐ valued
- ☐ worthy

Introduce Your Selfie/ Identity Slides

Grade Levels K–12

Target Competency

- Relationship Skills

Integrated Competencies

- Self-Awareness
- Self-Management
- Social Awareness

Sample Identity Slide

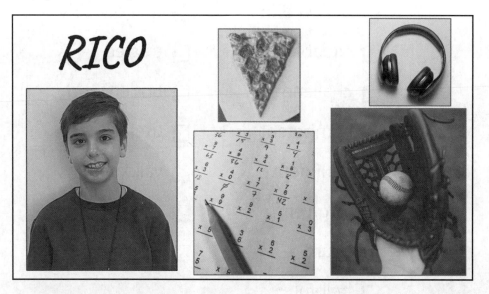

Purpose

Students share about themselves to build connections with their classmates and the teacher.

Materials

- Google Slides™ or PowerPoint®
- example of an Identity Slide
- *Introduce Your Selfie Planner* (page 154)
- sentence frames written on chart paper or on the board

Procedure

Note: This activity can be done in two parts. In Part 1, students design their Identity Slides. In Part 2, students view one another's slides and ask questions.

Part 1

1. Explain that your classroom is a community and that relationships develop when individuals get to know one another.

2. Share your own Identity Slide as an example.

3. Distribute the *Introduce Your Selfie Planner* and review it with students.

4. Have students create their own digital slides using the planner, working on a shared Google Slides™ deck or in PowerPoint®. If students are working in PowerPoint®, they can send their completed slide to you.

Part 2

1. Compile the slides into one deck or presentation.

2. Present the slides to the class.

3. Invite students to ask questions about their classmates' slides, using sentence frames as needed.

4. Students respond to the student reflection questions.

Specific Grade Level SEL Sentence Frames

Grades K–2

Differentiate the number of items that students share. Encourage students to use sentence frames.

> "What is your favorite _____?"

> "Why do you like _____?"

Grades 3–5

Differentiate the number of items that students share. Encourage students to use sentence frames and to generate their own questions.

"What do you like about _____?"

"Why do you like _____?"

"What does _____ mean to you?"

"I also like _____ because _____."

Grades 6–12

Emphasize the importance and value of diversity within the class. Students have the option of uploading video clips into their slides to introduce important people or places.

Encourage students to use sentence frames and to generate their own questions.

"One thing we have in common is _____."

"I am interested in why you chose _____. Can you tell me more?"

Student Reflection Questions

What did you learn about a classmate that you did not know before? What did you like about this activity?

Opportunities for Differentiation

- Integrate the arts by having students create Introduce Your Selfie posters.

- Revisit this activity by having students update their slides and reintroduce their selfies later in the year.

- Incorporate writing by having students write about their slides.

- Incorporate cooperative learning by having students discuss their slides in groups.

 Between Us

- This is a great opportunity to validate students' identities.

- Be sure that student names are pronounced correctly.

- Celebrate what students have in common and what makes them unique.

- This is meant to be a low-stress, fun activity. If students are reluctant to speak, provide support as needed.

- Feel free to have students generate some ideas of what to include on their slides.

Name: _____ Date: _____

Introduce Your Selfie Planner

Directions: Draw or write about what you like.

My Favorite Things

Food

Photo of Yourself

TV/YouTube®/ TikTok®

Sport

Color

Music

Book

Hobbies

Game/App

Subject

Holiday

126898—Social-Emotional Learning Starts with Us

SODAS (Situation, Options, Disadvantages, Advantages, Solution)

Grade Levels: 3–12

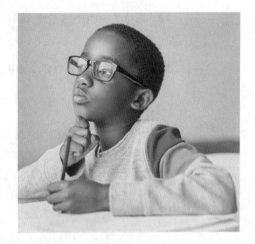

Target Competency
- Responsible Decision-Making

Integrated Competencies
- Self-Awareness
- Self-Management
- Social Awareness
- Relationship Skills

Purpose

Students learn how to solve problems, resolve conflicts, and make responsible decisions.

Materials

- *SODAS Chart* (page 158)
- sentence frames written on chart paper or on the board

Preparation

- Familiarize yourself with the SODAS framework and how to use the template.
- Select an example scenario to introduce SODAS.

Procedure

1. Explain the importance of responsible decision-making. Emphasize that decision-making is a process and takes practice to improve.

2. Introduce the SODAS acronym, and explain what it stands for (**S**ituation, **O**ptions, **D**isadvantages, **A**dvantages, **S**olution).

3. Ask students to help select a difficult decision to use as an example scenario.

4. Lead class through SODAS framework, thinking aloud as you identify the **S**ituation, three possible **O**ptions, the **D**isadvantages of each proposed option, and the **A**dvantages of each proposed option.

5. Review and evaluate each option. Ask students to weigh in on the process and the options.

6. Choose a **S**olution.

7. Ask students the reflection questions.

Specific Grade Level SEL Sentence Frames

Grades 3–5

At first, complete this activity as a whole group, and then have students work in cooperative learning groups. Later, if possible, have students complete this activity independently. Have them use sentence frames to justify their responses.

> "The advantages of this option are _____."

> "The disadvantages of this option are _____."

> "_____ is the best decision because _____."

Grades 6–12

Introduce ethical dilemmas to challenge your students to think critically about their own morals and ethics. For example, students can examine and discuss real-life situations from historical or current events. Have students cite evidence to justify their responses, and use sentence frames to elaborate on causes and effects.

> "The advantages of this option are _____."

> "The disadvantages of this option are _____."

> "_____ is a responsible decision because _____."

> "If _____ happens, then _____ will be the effect."

Student Reflection Questions

What did you find helpful about SODAS? What's one situation in your life where SODAS could be useful?

Opportunities for Differentiation

- Incorporate writing by having students write persuasive arguments for why their decision is the most responsible.

- Integrate the arts by having students act out or role-play scenarios.

- Support English learners by including visuals and written supports.

- Expand this activity by having students engage in a debate.

 # Between Us

- Use the gradual release of responsibility here. The goal is that students will be able to internalize the process and pause and consider their options before they act.

- Call out instances, or teachable moments, during the day when they can use SODAS.

- You can create a colorful poster of the SODAS chart to display in the classroom. Laminate it so it can be reused or so ideas can be added or changed.

Name: _____ Date: _____

SODAS Chart

Directions: Complete the chart to help make your decision.

SODAS

Situation • Options • Disadvantages • Advantages • Solution

Situation:

Option 1	Option 2	Option 3
Disadvantages	**Disadvantages**	**Disadvantages**
1.	1.	1.
2.	2.	2.
3.	3.	3.
Advantages	**Advantages**	**Advantages**
1.	1.	1.
2.	2.	2.
3.	3.	3.

Solution:

126898—Social-Emotional Learning Starts with Us

T-Chart

Grades Levels: K–2

Target Competency
- Responsible Decision-Making

Integrated Competencies
- Self-Management
- Self-Awareness
- Social Awareness
- Relationship Skills

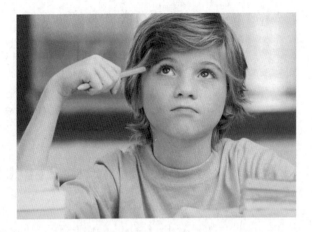

Purpose

Students learn to solve problems and make responsible decisions.

Materials

- T-chart template
- sentence frames written on chart paper or on the board

Preparation

- Familiarize yourself with a T-chart.
- Think of a scenario to introduce how to use a T-chart.

Procedure

1. Explain the importance of responsible decision-making.

2. Show how a T-chart is a graphic organizer that allows students to organize their thoughts and ideas.

3. Define the terms *pros* and *cons*.

4. Provide a sample scenario about a difficult situation, and think aloud to model how to use the T-chart to list the pros and cons of different possible solutions (see example on page 160).

5. Ask students to help you by adding more pros and cons.

6. Come to a consensus based on the identified pros and cons.

7. Ask students to respond to the reflection questions aloud.

Situation: Trying out for the school play

Pros	Cons
I could make friends.	People might make fun of me.
It is fun, and I would like an after-school activity.	I may not get a part and would be sad.
I will improve reading and public speaking.	It might take time away from playing with other friends.

Specific Grade Level SEL Sentence Frames

Grades K–2

At first, this activity can be completed as a group, and then students can gradually do it independently.

"I think a pro is _____."

"I feel _____ is a con because _____."

"I like the idea of _____ because _____."

"I do not like the idea of _____ because _____."

Student Reflection Questions

What is one thing you found helpful about using a T-chart? Name one situation in your life where a T-chart could be useful.

Opportunities for Differentiation

- Integrate the arts by having students act out or role-play scenarios.

- Vary the use of the T-chart using facts and opinions, strengths and areas of growth, or likes and dislikes.

- Support English learners by including visuals and other textual support in their home languages.

- Expand the lesson by having students justify their thinking.

- Have students complete their own T-charts before a writing assignment to brainstorm ideas.

 # Between Us

- As you guide students, make sure to model your thought process by thinking aloud.

- Validate students for their participation.

References

Ashoka United States. n.d. "Every Child Practicing Empathy." Accessed October 6, 2021. www.ashoka.org/en-us/focus/every-child-practicing-empathy/.

Aspen Institute. 2019. "From a Nation at Risk to a Nation at Hope: Recommendations from the National Commission on Social, Emotional, & Academic Development." nationathope.org/report-from-the-nation/.

Baldwin, James. n.d. "Remember this House." Unpublished manuscript.

Barmore, Peggy. 2021. "Schooling Has Changed Forever. Here's What Will Stay When Things Go Back to Normal." *The Hechinger Report*, March 16, 2021. hechingerreport.org/schooling-has-changed-forever-heres-what-will-stay-when-things-go-back-to-normal/.

Bennett, Jessica. 2020. "What if Instead of Calling People Out, We Called Them In?" *New York Times*, November 19, 2020. www.nytimes.com/2020/11/19/style/loretta-ross-smith-college-cancel-culture.html.

Brackett, Marc. 2019. *Permission to Feel: Unlocking the Power of Emotions to Help Our Kids, Ourselves, and Our Society Thrive*. New York: Celadon Books.

Brown, Adrienne M. 2017. *Emergent Strategy*. Chico, CA: AK Press.

Center for Healthy Minds. n.d. "What Is Neuroplasticity?" Accessed October 6, 2021. centerhealthyminds.org/feature/neuroplasticity.

Cherry, Kendra. 2020. "What Is the Negativity Bias?" *Verywell Mind*, April 29, 2020. www.verywellmind.com/negative-bias-4589618.

Collaborative for Academic, Social, and Emotional Learning (CASEL). 2019. "SEL 3 Signature Practices Playbook: A Tool that Supports Systemic SEL." *Guide to Schoolwide SEL*. schoolguide.casel.org/resource/three-signature-sel-practices-for-the-classroom.

Collaborative for Academic, Social, and Emotional Learning (CASEL). 2021. "Equity and SEL." *Guide to Schoolwide SEL*. schoolguide.casel.org/what-is-sel/equity-and-sel/.

Collaborative for Academic, Social, and Emotional Learning (CASEL). 2022. "SEL as a Lever for Equity and Excellence." drc.casel.org/sel-as-a-lever-for-equity/.

Collaborative for Academic, Social, and Emotional Learning (CASEL). n.d. "Fundamentals of SEL." Accessed September 28, 2021. casel.org/fundamentals-of-sel/.

Comas-Diaz, Lilian, Gordon N. Hall, and Helen A. Neville. 2019. "Racial Trauma: Theory, Research, and Healing: Introduction to the Special Issue." *American Psychology* 74, no. 1 (January): 1–5. pubmed.ncbi.nlm.nih.gov/30652895/.

Cranston, Amy. 2019. *Creating Social and Emotional Learning Environments*. Huntington Beach, CA: Shell Education.

Darling-Hammond, Linda, Pamela Cantor, Laura E. Hernández, Abby Schachner, Sara Plasencia, Christina Theokas, and Elizabeth Tijerina. 2021. *Design Principles for Schools: Putting the Science of Learning and Development into Action*. Palo Alto, CA: Learning Policy Institute; New York: Turnaround for Children. k12.designprinciples.org/sites/default/files/SoLD_Design_Principles_REPORT.pdf

Desautels, Lori. 2021. "Bad Behavior or Nervous System Response: A New Lens for Discipline." *Alliance Against Seclusion and Restraint*, February 20, 2021. endseclusion.org/2021/02/20/bad-behavior-or-nervous-system-response/.

Dewey, John. 1933. *How We Think: A Restatement of the Relation of Reflective Thinking to the Educative Process*. Chicago: Henry Regnery.

Doran, G. T. 1981. "There's a S.M.A.R.T. Way to Write Management's Goals and Objectives." *Management Review* 70 (11): 35–36.

Dweck, Carol S. 2006. *Mindset: The New Psychology of Success*. New York: Random House.

Eisler, Melissa. 2019. "Explaining the Difference Between Mindfulness and Meditation." *Chopra*, August 27, 2019. chopra.com/articles/explaining-the-difference-between-mindfulness-meditation.

Flanagan, Linda. 2017. "How Parents Can Help Kids Develop a Sense of Purpose." *MindShift*, May 18, 2017. www.kqed.org/mindshift/48013/how-parents-can-help-kids-develop-a-sense-of-purpose.

Frankl, Viktor E. 1946. *Man's Search for Meaning*. Boston: Beacon Press.

Gay, Geneva. 2000. "Culturally Responsive Teaching in Special Education for Ethnically Diverse Students: Setting the Stage." *International Journal of Qualitative Studies in Education* 15 (6): 613–629.

Hammond, Zaretta. 2015. *Culturally Responsive Teaching and the Brain*. Thousand Oaks, CA: Corwin.

Herman, Keith C., Jal'et Hickmon, and Wendy M. Reinke. 2018. "Empirically Derived Profiles of Teacher Stress, Burnout, Self-Efficacy, and Coping and Associated Student Outcomes." *Journal of Positive Behavior Interventions* 20 (2): 90–100. doi.org/10.1177/1098300717732066.

Hollie, Sharroky. 2018. *Culturally and Linguistically Responsive Teaching and Learning*. 2nd ed. Huntington Beach, CA: Shell Education.

Irvine, Jacqueline J., and Willis D. Hawley. 2011. "Culturally Responsive Pedagogy: An Overview of Research on Student Outcomes." Paper presented at Teaching Tolerance: A Project of the Southern Poverty Law Center: Culturally Responsive Teaching Awards Celebration, Pew Conference Center, Washington, DC, December 2011.

References

Jagers, Robert J., Deborah Rivas-Drake, and Teresa Borowski. 2018. "Equity & Social and Emotional Learning: A Cultural Analysis." *Measuring SEL: Using Data to Inspire Practice* (Special Issue Series).

Jones, Stephanie, Rick Weissbourd, Suzanne Bouffard, Jennifer Kahn, and Trisha Ross Anderson. n.d. "How to Build Empathy and Strengthen Your School Community." *Making Caring Common Project.* Cambridge, MA: Harvard Graduate School of Education. Accessed October 6, 2021. mcc.gse.harvard.edu/resources-for-educators/how-build-empathy-strengthen-school-community.

Kabat-Zinn, Jon. 1994. *Wherever You Go, There You Are: Mindfulness Meditation in Everyday Life.* New York: Hachette Books.

Kurtz, Holly, Alex Harwin, and Olivia Blomstrom. 2019. "Safety and Social-Emotional Learning: Results of a National Survey." *Education Week Research Center.* Accessed September 20, 2021. epe.brightspotcdn.com/65/30/761a98ea490a90b8bcac85bf7724/safety-and-sel-national-survey-education-week-research-center-2019.pdf.

Ladson-Billings, Gloria. 1994. *The Dreamkeepers.* San Francisco: Jossey-Bass.

Ladson-Billings, Gloria. 2014. "Culturally Relevant Pedagogy 2.0: a.k.a. the Remix." *Harvard Educational Review* 84 (1): 74–84.

Lee, Laura. 2019. "The Benefits of Teaching Ethical Dilemmas." *Edutopia*, July 18, 2019. www.edutopia.org/article/benefits-teaching-ethical-dilemmas

Leo, Pam. 2007. *Connection Parenting: Parenting through Connection Instead of Coercion, through Love Instead of Fear.* 2nd ed. Deadwood, OR: Wyatt-MacKenzie Publishing, Inc.

Lopez, Shane, and Preety Sidhu. 2013. "U.S. Teachers Love Their Lives but Struggle in the Workplace." Gallup poll, March 28, 2013. news.gallup.com/poll/161516/teachers-love-lives-struggle-workplace.aspx.

Maynard, Nathan, and Brad Weinstein. 2019. *Hacking School Discipline: 9 Ways to Create a Culture of Empathy and Responsibility Using Restorative Justice.* Highland Heights, OH: Times 10 Publications.

Mindful Schools. n.d. "Research on Mindfulness." Accessed October 6, 2021. www.mindfulschools.org/about-mindfulness/research-on-mindfulness/.

News Bureau, University of Missouri. 2018. "More Than 9 in 10 Elementary School Teachers Feel Highly Stressed, MU Study Finds." News release, April 24, 2018. munewsarchives.missouri.edu/news-releases/2018/0424-more-than-9-in-10-elementary-school-teachers-feel-highly-stressed-mu-study-finds/index.html.

Perry, Bruce D., and Oprah Winfrey. 2021. *What Happened to You? Conversations on Trauma, Resilience, and Healing.* New York: Flatiron Books.

Pink, Daniel. 2011. *Drive: The Surprising Truth About What Motivates Us.* New York: Riverhead.

Psychology Today Staff. n.d. "Gratitude." *Psychology Today.* Accessed October 6, 2021. www.psychologytoday.com/us/basics/gratitude.

Rockwell, Jill. 2019. "Social and Emotional Learning Part 5 of 5: Responsible Decision-Making." *The Connecting Link*, February 18, 2019. www.connectinglink.com/blog/responsible_decision-making.

Ruiz, Don Jose. 2018. *Wisdom of the Shamans: What the Ancient Masters Can Teach Us About Love and Life.* San Antonio, TX: Hierophant Publishing.

Schlund, Justina, Robert J. Jagers, and Melissa Schlinger. 2020. *Emerging Insights on Advancing Social and Emotional Learning (SEL) as a Lever for Equity and Excellence.* Chicago: CASEL. casel.org/wp-content/uploads/2020/08/CASEL-Equity-Insights-Report.pdf.

Simmons, Dena. 2019. "How to Be an Antiracist Educator." *ASCD*, October 1, 2019. www.ascd.org/publications/newsletters/education-update/oct19/vol61/num10/How-to-Be-an-Antiracist-Educator.aspx.

Simmons, Dena N., Marc A. Brackett, and Nancy Adler. 2018. *Applying an Equity Lens to Social, Emotional, and Academic Development.* University Park, PA: Edna Bennett Pierce Prevention Research Center, Pennsylvania State University. www.prevention.psu.edu/uploads/files/rwjf446338-EquityLens.pdf.

Stanford Children's Health. n.d. "Understanding the Teen Brain." Accessed October 6, 2021. www.stanfordchildrens.org/en/topic/default?id=understanding-the-teen-brain-1-3051.

Tennant, Jaclyn E., Michelle K. Demaray, Christine K. Malecki, Melissa N. Terry, Michael Clary, and Nathan Elzinga. 2015. "Students' Ratings of Teacher Support and Academic and Social-Emotional Well-Being." *School Psychology Quarterly* 30 (4): 494–512. psycnet.apa.org/record/2014-56438-001.

Wallace, David F. 2005. "This Is Water." Commencement speech, Kenyon College.

Waterford.org. 2019. "Why Strong Teacher Relationships Lead to Student Engagement and a Better School Environment." www.waterford.org/education/teacher-student-relationships/.

Whitlock, Janis. n.d. "Cultivating a Sense of Purpose in Youth." Presentation for the Bronfenbrenner Center for Translational Research, Ithaca, NY. Accessed October 6, 2021. www.actforyouth.net/resources/pd/pd14-purpose.pdf.

Yancey-Bragg, N'Dea. 2020. "What Is Systemic Racism? Here's What It Means and How You Can Help Dismantle It." *USA Today*, January 29, 2020. www.usatoday.com/story/news/nation/2020/06/15/systemic-racism-what-does-mean/5343549002/.

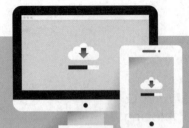

Digital Resources

Accessing the Digital Resources

The digital resources can be downloaded by following these steps:

1. Go to **www.tcmpub.com/digital**

2. Enter the ISBN, which is located on the back cover of the book, into the appropriate field on the website.

3. Respond to the prompts using the book to view your account and available digital content.

4. Choose the digital resources you would like to download. You can download all the files at once, or you can download a specific group of files.

ISBN:
978-1-0876-4918-4

Please note: Some files provided for download have large file sizes. Download times for these larger files will vary based on your download speed.

 ## Contents of the Digital Resources

You will find digital versions of the student activity pages in this book. These digital resources offer greater flexibility and accessibility than the print resources alone. You can use them on interactive whiteboards, for virtual sessions, in LMS platforms, and more!